The EAT RIGHT FEEL GOOD LOSE WEIGHT HAVE FUN COOK BOOK

"You Won't Be Hungry"

Sherry Granader
with foreword by Lou Ferrigno

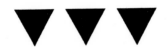

LARKSDALE
HOUSTON

The
  Eat Right
    Feel Good
      Lose Weight
        Have Fun
          Cookbook

Editor: Shelia Stewart Darst

Design: Joann Thurman

Graphics: Costner Graphics

Cover Photography: J. Pamela Photography, Inc.

Food Photgraphy: J. Pamela Photography, Inc.

ISBN # 0-89896-215-3

LARKSDALE

Printed in the United States of America

Dedication

To my husband,
Dan Granader, my best critic and supporter,
and the best taste-tester around!

To my parents,
June and Bill Halliday, who taught me how
to handle food, entertain with ease, and who
support my every endeavor with
much love and enthusiasm!

To my in-laws,
Sylvia and Harry Granader, who love my cooking,
especially my coffee, and who choose to eat at our
home instead of going out when they visit!

Camp-Mak-A-Dream

Part of the proceeds from the sale of this cookbook will be given to The Children's Oncology Camp Foundation in Gold Creek, Montana.

Children's Oncology Camp Foundation, founded by Harry and Sylvia Granader, Birmingham, Michigan, was created to provide children with cancer and other dreaded diseases, a normal summer camp experience.

The Foundation is a non-profit volunteer organization and all donations are tax deductible. The camp is called Camp-Mak-A-Dream, to be built in Gold Creek, Montana, and all funding provided through donations is entirely free of charge for all children. All kids should experience the exciting activity of summer camp. Unfortunately, medical and financial circumstances have often kept children with cancer from embarking on such adventures. Happily, camp for these children is now a reality.

Camp-Mak-A-Dream is a special camp which will give children with cancer the opportunity to engage in a wide variety of recreation activities and learning experiences, such as fishing, nature hiking, horseback riding, arts and crafts, volleyball, soccer, archery, and other camp activities with trained instructors to supervise.

Camp-Mak-A-Dream carefully meets the camper's medical needs by supplementing a regular camp staff with professional pediatric oncology personnel.

Camp-Mak-A-Dream combines fun with proper health care for each child. Medical personnel will be available at all times to administer routine chemotherapy, perform necessary blood counts, and handle any emergencies.

While love and protection are natural responses, there is a tendency for children with cancer to be over-protected by parents and friends. The kids, themselves, often need the freedom to romp, play, and learn on their own.

This camp will give a child an important chance to gain independence, play, make new friends, laugh a lot, and just have fun.

The
EAT RIGHT
FEEL GOOD
LOSE WEIGHT
HAVE FUN
COOK BOOK
**"You Won't
Be Hungry"**

Sherry Granader
with foreword by Lou Ferrigno

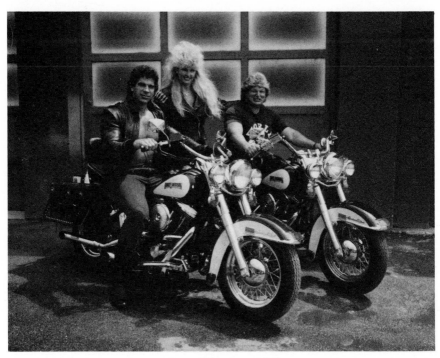

Lou, Sherry, and Dan

FOREWORD

I recall the first time I met Dan and Sherry Granader. I had been invited to Houston, Texas for the grand opening of their World Gym. It's rare to meet a couple and hit it off from the beginning, but we did. And we have been friends since. After the successful opening of the gym and the autograph sessions, we spent the rest of the weekend working out together and having a lot of fun! We have the same interests and the same family values. Dan has a wonderful sense of humor, and Sherry is one of the busiest people I know!

Sherry and I did a lot of photo sessions with a group of models that appeared in Muscle and Fitness Magazine. After the photo sessions, I didn't see Sherry for five or six months, but when I did, I was pleasantly surprised to see how she had begun to change her physique. With much determination, she totally changed her eating habits, and I saw her making better eating choices in restaurants. She began to include weight training and aerobics in her workouts at least four days a week.

Sherry is a wonderful cook and enjoys cooking for a crowd. On visits to our home, she has prepared some of her low-fat recipes for my family's approval. Her style of cooking shows that proper diet is one of the major keys to having a successful body, but proper diet doesn't have to include dull and boring meals.

I appreciate Dan and Sherry's support and friendship and look forward to many years of fun times together, whenever possible. Too bad they don't live in California! But Sherry is blazing a healthy nutritional trail in Texas with her Low-Fat Cooking Schools, her Weight Management Seminars, and now with this cookbook. I wish her well, and I wish you: Good Eating...Good Health ... Granader Style!

Lou Ferrigno

Photos

A special thank you to photographers Pam Culpepper of J. Pamela Photography, Inc. and Ian Martin and Todd Pencarinha who graciously took pictures with the reward of eating all the food as soon as the picture was taken! Also, a special thank you to Joann Thurman for spending the day helping me arrange all my props!

PART I

PART I

Table of Contents

1 Eat Right...Don't Diet

Let's face it. Dieting is a dreaded endeavor, and according to most statistics, an expensive, wasted effort. Most diets fail most dieters. Most dieters fail most diets. When hunger signals, the body is in need and must not be ignored. However, most diets imply starvation, not fulfillment. To some people, hunger is a sign of feeling guilty rather than a time to fuel the body and enjoy good food.

Throw out the diet, not the food!

By learning to eat sensibly, by developing motivation, by changing lifestyles, and by exercising, weight loss can be an attainable goal.

Do those things sound like lofty ideals prescribed by every fitness expert and health guru? Probably, yes; however, with nutritional knowledge comes understanding. Strive to be wise consumers, informed cooks, nutrition experts, and fitness seekers. Don't throw out everything in the kitchen and start from scratch. That's unrealistic. Simply, learn the principles of low-fat substitution and learn to balance protein and carbohydrates.

When most people go on a diet, the first things thrown out are the carbohydrates. Potatoes, bread, and pasta become the enemy when actually, these foods give energy, and when balanced with protein, can lead to weight loss.

Sixty percent of each meal should contain carbohydrates. Carbohydrates include vegetables, fruits, grains, and sugars. Refined carbohydrates (sugars and starches) should be eaten with care. Very simply, add more complex carbohydrates to your diet. Choose a fruit or vegetable and a rice, pasta, bread, cereal, or potato.

Twenty percent of each meal should include protein. Protein is needed to develop and maintain muscle tone. Whatever protein is left in the body, after digestion and use, is eliminated through waste products.

Twenty percent of each meal needs to include fat. A certain amount of fat is necessary to keep hair shiny and skin lubricated and youthful looking. Fat is also necessary for proper liver and kidney function. However, measure fat content carefully. Use only polyunsaturated or monounsaturated fat. This will not only help with weight loss but will help control cholesterol levels.

This combination of foods, equaling ten grams of fat per meal, totals 30 grams of daily fat. This appropriate combination of foods is the key to weight loss.

Most diets are fads. People will lose weight, but the same people will become a yo-yo statistic. They lose the weight, then gain it back. Americans annually spend over $30 million dollars a year on products to help lose weight. The United States is a fat-conscious society without consciousness for change. Why spend millions on products or ways not to eat, when food is the answer to successful, healthy eating habits?

Even though I had been exercising, doing aerobics, and work-ing with weights, it was not until I developed the Eat Right...Don't Diet program that I lost over twenty pounds and almost three dress sizes.

Weight training, aerobics, and exercise will not give proper benefits unless eating right techniques are learned. Eating right starts with cooking right. Healthy food preparation must begin at home.

I love to eat and fortunately, love to cook. Through trial and error, I have learned to cook tasty, low-calorie meals which are, most of all, easy to prepare. I do not have degrees in nutrition to make me an expert. I have become a self-taught expert. I started by reading everything I could about diet, nutrition, and fitness. I memorized charts categorizing food according to fat content and calories. Then, I got in the kitchen and began to adapt recipes to be low calorie and low fat.

The fat in most recipes can be cut in half very easily. Eliminate oil, butter, margarine, mayonnaise, and sour cream. Sugar and salt can be deleted from most recipes. Finding alternatives is the answer! Add flavored extracts to recipes to make food appealing to both taste and sight. If food doesn't look appetizing on the plate or table, it won't be eaten.

Food should be a whole experience satisfying all senses.

Food presentation is very important. Make food look opulent by using the Sunday silver, a lace tablecloth, and fine china. Dress up the table with fresh flowers and napkin rings.

Egg whites can do everything the whole egg can do. Use two egg whites for every whole egg in a recipe. Egg whites are a major source of protein and can be made to look and taste the way eggs are expected to look and taste by using spices and flavorings. All fat in an egg is contained in the yolk. Because of today's lifestyles, food preparation must be quick and easy. Otherwise, dependency on traditional cooking methods and recipes will cause a return to high-calorie, high-fat, preparation habits. If it isn't easy, don't deal with it.

Certainly, I advocate fresh first; however, if there isn't available time to grow, purchase, or find fresh fruits, herbs, and vegetables, frozen is fine. The microwave oven is one of the low-fat cook's best friends. Frying is unnecessary with the microwave. Oils and lard are made obsolete.

Grilling is the best way to cook meats. If possible, invest in an outdoor grill or indoor gas grill. Fat from meat drops down and burns up. The meat does not sit in or absorb any fat.

Most people on traditional diets starve themselves to shed the pounds. Depriving the body of needed nutrients only leads to poor health. Dieters develop headaches, muscle pain, and weakness. The energy level drops dramatically because of lacking nourishment. Dieters suffer from a form of withdrawal with typical, adverse symptoms.

Exercise at this point will do little good to help the dieter. Exercise must be a partner in weight loss.

Like food, exercise must be enjoyed!

Dieting to lose weight without exercising or exercising to lose weight without dieting will not accomplish set goals. These two aspects must work together. The program must be balanced, like everything in life. Also, that balance is different for each person.

Naturally, I advocate exercise programs offered in gyms. Weight training and aerobic classes can be developed for the individual. Fitness experts and trainers are available to offer advice. Proper equipment is available. Plus, working out in a group is fun! The atmosphere is social and cheerful, if the gym programs are non-competitive and individually structured.

If a gym facility is inaccessible, either by locale or for special reasons, classes are offered at local schools, colleges, YMCA's, and churches. Tapes and records are available that would help with home fitness programs. Television offers beneficial, exercise programs. Walking for exercise is wonderful! The most important thing is to have fun and be consistent, whatever form the exercise program takes. The amount of exercise each person needs will vary; however, a program which features a forty minute workout three or four days a week is a basic beginning.

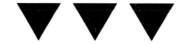

2 Sherry's Personal Philosophy

In September, 1981, my husband and I moved to Houston, Texas from Michigan to open a fast food restaurant. Within eighteen months, we acquired five fast food establishments, extra pounds, an insane schedule, and too much stress.

By 1982, we were managing seven restaurants with over 700 employees. This meant eating on the run and usually eating the fast food we served. Then, fast food always was high in fat and usually fried.

Although I had been involved in sports growing up and in college, the schedule of owning and managing seven restaurants severely limited my exercising. My husband had always worked out since playing collegiate football and had competed nationally in power lifting. But even he found our schedule to be disruptive to a structured, fitness regimen.

To relieve tension and stress and to help lose the weight I had gained, my husband suggested I try low-impact aerobic and body sculpting classes.

After working the lunch rush in drive-thru, I decided I was ready to do something for myself to help myself. The classes were wonderful, and one instructor became my mentor.

I loved what the exercises did for my body, and I appreciated my new outlook on life. I was dealing with stress much better, and I developed strength and tone without doing high-impact aerobics.

With guidance and expertise from my fitness instructor, I structured my own routines to music and began teaching a body sculpting class. Many women enjoyed my class so much that they continue to take the class to this day.

As my husband and I became more involved with gyms, we noticed what we called the tough guy/sweat sock mentality directing the management of most such fitness establishments. The equipment was old, in need of repair, or inappropriate.

Cleanliness was lacking. Families were not welcome. Competitive training was stressed.

We decided that if the management principles of the fast food restaurant business were applied to a gym, an establishment could be developed which was clean, well-equipped, family-oriented, well-lighted, safe, cheerful, and non-competitive in atmosphere.

We applied for a World Gym franchise and opened our first facility in a suburb of Houston, Texas. Our fifth location will open this year and expansion to Dallas is planned for the near future.

After selling the restaurants and opening the gym, I began teaching more classes. My husband and I changed our lifestyle, exercise habits, schedule, and menu.

I became fascinated with the nutritional advice given by experts. Most nutritional information was incomplete, confusing, and misleading. Thank goodness, food labeling is being changed by the government so that the ordinary consumer can understand nutritional values and become more knowledgeable. Within a year, new FDA guidelines will be established to help consumers make more intelligent choices. Also, with increased nutritional awareness, more and more products are being developed which are lower in fat or reduced in calories. Food manufacturers are making substitutions and redoing traditional mass market recipes.

I developed a personal philosophy about eating, food consumption, and exercise, and I began searching for the quickest, easiest, most low-fat way to prepare familiar meals. I started by changing well-loved, family recipes from high-fat, high-calorie meals into low-fat delights. I remembered recipes from a favorite Michigan tea room and adapted these to be part of my new balanced lifestyle.

Although I was exercising and teaching aerobics, it was not until I began low-fat substitution and balanced protein/carbohydrate eating that I shed pounds. With the program I developed for myself, I was actually eating more, including snacks, and losing weight. And I felt really terrific! I was not hungry. I was happy. Instead of counting calories and watching the scale, I was reading labels and learning low-fat, substitution techniques.

Several members in the gym could not believe the difference in my physical appearance and wanted to know how I had lost the weight. I talked to these members individually and tried to explain the program one on one. However, so many people wanted to know about my philosophy that I put together a plan that included four sessions to teach women how to eat right without dieting, and how to work out to get desired results. The first session concerned nutrition and the next three were workout sessions in the gym.

Word spread, and before I knew it, I was booked solid, training eight women a day including weekends. Suddenly, there was a waiting list for my classes. It has been crazy; however, the satisfaction I have received, from helping others learn to eat right and still lose weight, has been most stimulating.

My teaching program has expanded to include not only nutrition and exercise, but shopping tips and the recipes I have developed. I put up a poster with an 8 x 10 glossy of myself in a leotard with the catch phrase, "Lose Weight! You Won't Be Hungry! Have Fun! Recipes Included! By Appointment Only! Ask for Sherry!" To say the least, I could not call people back quickly enough. To date, I have personally trained over 200 women.

While teaching exercise and nutrition to my clients, questions naturally came up about food and recipes. I started sharing experiences, opinions, recipes, and hints. From that, Sherry's Low-Fat Cooking School opened.

Classes are held once a month for two hours at the Sports Cafe in the gym. Students eat everything they cook. Each student receives the recipes of the day as well as general nutrition tips for good eating. The grocery shopping and table decorations are done early so as many recipes as possible can be prepared during class. Students enjoy sparkling cider in champagne glasses while covering aspects of general nutrition. Then, the class adjourns to the kitchen to cook the low-fat meals and eat everything.

Typical topics covered are "Low-Fat, Low-Calorie, Quick Main Dishes," "Low-Fat Cookies and Muffins," "Low-Fat Gourmet Cooking—European Style," "Decadent Desserts for Cheat Day." It is so much fun to mingle with people who like to eat, cook, and get fit while having a good time!

Since the opening of the low-fat cooking schools last spring, I have been swamped with requests for interviews. An article about the school appeared in the November, 1991 *Fitness Management* magazine. Several local papers have featured my cooking school and programs. Obviously, people are fascinated by low-fat cooking, fat substitution, weight loss, and the fitness programs which I have developed.

After reading the article in *Fitness Management* magazine, a representative from Hickam Air Force Base in Hawaii called me. He asked if I would come to the islands and conduct my low-fat cooking seminars on the base. He explained that fitness facilities were available to service men and their families on all bases, but information about good nutrition and eating right was lacking. Arrangements have been made for me to conduct these classes in Hawaii. Aloha!

Also, I have appeared with Lee Haney, Mr. Olympia, on the cable television channel, ESPN. He was in Houston to train with Evander Holyfield, heavyweight champion, at one of our facilities and asked if I would fill in on his program for one of his regulars off on leave.

I have conducted fitness and nutrition seminars for Shell Oil employees and the Association of Business and Professional Women.

Everyone seems to be getting into the Eat Right habit!

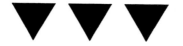

3 Setting Up The Eat Right Program

The right combination of food is the key to success when beginning the new low-fat eating and fitness program:

Sixty percent of each meal needs to include carbohydrates;

Twenty percent of each meal should include protein;

Twenty percent of each meal will include fat.

This combination of foods totals 30 grams of fat for the day which means that during each meal 10 grams of fat can be consumed.

For example:

One boneless, skinless chicken breast, grilled equals 6 grams of fat.

One baked potato served plain with non-fat toppings equals 3 grams of fat.

One serving of steamed vegetables served with flavorings, pepper, or seasonings equals 1 gram of fat.

The total meal will equal 10 grams of fat.

This combination of foods must be understood to enjoy a complete meal, lose weight, and feel great. High-protein diets alone fail because the balance of correct carbohydrates is not considered. It is this balance of proper protein and carbohydrates, with low-fat cooking, which will take the weight off. Add exercise, and good health can be enjoyed!

If just a salad is eaten for lunch, hunger will attack in about two hours or less! At this point, the body is demanding something to fill a need, and a fattening snack is what most people find to be the solution to the hunger. As long as the suggested balance of foods is eaten at each meal, hunger will not dominate. Healthy, low-fat snacks are allowed on this program as long as the total grams of fat does not go over 30 grams per day. Keeping within ten grams fat per meal will allow weight loss and maintenance for life.

Exercise, aerobics, or weight training will play an important role in the daily regimen. Exercise of any sort will elevate the body temperature. This allows the body to burn up calories and burn off body fat. Exercise strengthens muscles and bones to help prevent osteoporosis.

When I first meet with a new client, I have her outline a typical day including when meals are taken, where meals are taken, if meals are taken alone or with other people, and what types of food are eaten at each meal. Snacks are discussed and favorite restaurant meals noted.

I have found that most of my clients skip breakfast or have only toast and coffee. Breakfast is a critical meal. It sets the tone for the whole day. If high-energy foods are not eaten at breakfast, the body will demand something later in the day which usually comes in the form of a high-calorie, high-fat snack at mid-morning. A salad at lunch is not the answer to losing weight. This causes hunger and body distress which leads to non-nutritious snacking. After not eating properly all day, a client might binge at dinner or be the prudent dieter and have only chicken or fish at supper. Either supper plan will fail.

This type of eating plan always fails a dieter. My clients found that instead of losing weight, they were developing health problems. They would suffer from a lack of energy, headaches, muscle pain, lethargy, high blood pressure, or stress-related disorders. The frustration of being on a diet without success can lead to tension, depression, and low self-esteem.

The right combination of foods at each meal is critical for the development of a healthy eating plan. Everyone is different, and each plan will have differences to accommodate that individual's needs.

You really do have to make time to eat!

Think of your body as a computer. It only functions as well as what is entered. If you do not enter enough information or the wrong information, the computer will malfunction. Your body is the same! You must feed your body the right foods and enough food to keep it running at optimum levels.

Quick, low-fat meals, which stay with you for at least three hours, are the key to preparation. If I can do it with my hectic schedule, so can you! It can be so easy and fun! I want you to look forward to your meals and not feel guilty because you are hungry. You must eat! But eat right!

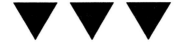

4   Sherry's Low-Fat Program

Eliminating the egg yolk from eggs is critical. All fat in eggs is stored in the yolk. Learning to cook with and eat just the white on an egg is an important part of the plan. Egg whites are a significant source of protein.

Remember the formula. For every whole egg, use two egg whites. Whenever a recipe calls for three eggs, substitute six egg whites. Egg separators can be purchased at most hardware or general merchandise stores to make the separation easier and eliminate the risk of any egg yolk escaping into the food.

Some people look at me like I am crazy when I ask them to eat three or four egg whites when they are just starting a new, exercise program. Five or six egg whites need to be consumed every morning at breakfast if that person has been on a weight training program for any length of time.

There are many delicious and quick ways to prepare egg whites. This can be a fun, new breakfast food!

One way to prepare egg whites quickly is with an egg poacher. Begin by filling the saucepan half-full with water and set on high heat. Spray poacher cups with vegetable spray, and drop each egg into a cup. Season with seasoned salt, which adds color and gives the egg a wonderful flavor. Cover. By the time the eggs are cooked to the hard-boiled stage, the potato will be done. Yes! Potatoes are not only legal but an important source of carbohydrates.

I use new, red potatoes the size of my fist in most recipes. Microwave the scrubbed potato for two minutes. Remove and cut into squares. Drop into a skillet coated with vegetable spray and cook on high heat. Flavor with seasoned salt and onion powder.

Scrambling egg whites for an omelet is another delicious way to prepare eggs for breakfast. Separate the egg white from the yolk, and scramble the whites in a skillet coated with vegetable spray. Add tomatoes, green peppers, onions, mushrooms, or

26

picante sauce. The eggs will be low-fat, low-calorie, filling, colorful, and nutritious. Top the scrambled egg whites with non-fat, cheddar cheese, and Molly McButter bacon flavored seasoning. This is a treat!.

In addition to the egg whites and potato, have a piece of toast with spreadable fruit (available in the jelly and jam section of most grocery stores). No butter allowed on toast!

Remember the adage, "It's better to eat the fruit than drink the juice," so, have a piece of fruit with breakfast. Plums and strawberries are the preferred fruits to eat, when dieting, because they emulsify fat.

Digestion of certain foods will increase the metabolic rate at different levels. For every one hundred calories of carbohydrates consumed, a ten per cent metabolic increase can be expected. It takes more energy to digest oats than it does to digest yogurt. Same thing applies to fruit. It takes more energy to digest plums and strawberries than it does to digest bananas.

Many people must have coffee in the morning; however, limit coffee intake to no more than two cups. Sweeten lightly with sugar. Artificial sweeteners may increase hunger. Because it is not known how these sweeteners are processed by the body, use sugar. Remember that it takes a full, twenty-four hours for caffeine to be eliminated from the system. Drink water the rest of the day. Also, try to drink a glass of water with your cup of coffee – this will help curb the craving for another cup! Eventually you will find yourself reaching for the water instead of the coffee because it feels better to the body.

Breakfast is the time to take a multivitamin and mineral supplement. Learn to read labels and compare.

A high-potency vitamin and mineral supplement must be taken daily if working out more than three or four times a week. The calcium and iron are essential when exercising.

If the morning is rushed, substitute one serving of cream of wheat or oatmeal for the potato, egg, and toast. Flavor the cereal with cinnamon, raisins, and vanilla extract (1 teaspoon) before microwaving. Do not add milk or butter.

Three hours after breakfast, it's snack time, and one of my favorites was developed by nutritionist, Keith Kline. Use 8 ounces of any flavor light yogurt. Add 1/3 cup raw oats and 2 tablespoons raisins. Blend until well mixed. The oats emulsify fat in the body, and the snack is very filling.

Since most people rush through lunch, I include fast food restaurants on the eat-right plan. Most of these restaurants now offer a grilled chicken sandwich, which can even be ordered in the drive-thru and eaten in the car. This is not ideal, but consideration must be given to lifestyles. Order the sandwich plain or with lettuce, tomato, mustard, pickles, ketchup, barbecue sauce, or onions. Do not have the special sauces, mayonnaise, cheese, or bacon.

With the grilled chicken sandwich, order a small salad with low-fat dressing OR a plain, baked potato. Keep Molly McButter flavorings with you in your car. With the selection of flavorings offered, the potato will be loaded with taste, without the fat.

It is now 4 o'clock in the afternoon and time for another snack. Have frozen, light yogurt without toppings. Fruit is a filling, quick energy snack food. The point here is to eat the snack. Make time. Have a snack. This is not an option.

The idea of eating dinner before six in the evening is unrealistic because of most people's hectic schedule. It is what is eaten after six that adds weight.

With the new, nutritional awareness, thankfully, more low-fat food choices are available. Turkey and chicken can now be purchased ground or skinless and boneless. Several manufacturers have developed marinated chicken and turkey breasts. These have four to six grams of fat per piece. Choose teriyaki, tomato herb, lemon herb, or barbeque. Stay away from the Mexican and Italian Bleu Cheese flavors, because they contain 10 to 14 grams of fat per serving.

As substitute for regular beef, I recommend buffalo meat. Buffalo has fifty percent more protein than beef with forty percent less fat. Buffalo can be substituted in any recipe which calls for beef. Make buffalo burgers, stuffed bell pepper with buffalo, spaghetti sauce with buffalo, buffalo meatloaf ... the possibilities are endless.

Fish is another alternative for dinner. Grill tuna steaks on open flame of a gas grill or broil in the oven with lemon and herbs.

Veal is another good, low-fat meat source for dinner. Grill the veal and have the sauce on the side.

Be creative with selections and recipes. Chicken, fish, and turkey don't have to be tiresome!

After selecting the protein source for dinner, chose the carbohydrate. If baked potatoes have become boring, try any of the rice mixes available. However, when the mixing directions say to add butter...DON'T.

Pasta is an excellent, complex carbohydrate for dinner selection. Stay away from the stuffed ravioli. Add a salad topped with non-fat dressing or a steamed vegetable.

Don't just have a baked potato and think this helps the weight loss cause. A protein source, a carbohydrate, and the allowed fat must be included to have a balanced meal.

For dessert, a piece of fruit is quick and sweet, or try one of my delicious, dessert recipes to end an excellent meal without guilt.

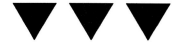

5 Eat Right and Still Celebrate

The best way to eat right and not gain weight during those holiday times is to eat as many meals daily as would normally be consumed. Don't try to starve all day and think gorging will be legal later at that big, family dinner.

You'll feel much better afterward if you don't skip any meals during the holiday seasons. A hearty meal at dinner can still be consumed if the prescribed intake of fat, protein, and carbohydrates is adhered to according to schedule. You won't need to eat as much food to celebrate, and your body will thank you later! Concentrate on the festivities with family and friends instead of focusing only on food.

It takes more energy to break down protein in the body, before it is stored as fat, than it does any other nutrient. Carbohydrates are needed for energy and are either quickly burned or deposited as fat. If fat is eliminated from the diet, more protein and carbohydrates can be eaten with less risk of adding fat to the body.

If something fattening is consumed, it will seem that the feeling of fullness is maintained longer. This occurs because the breakdown process of the protein and carbohydrates, plus fat, takes longer. If a low-fat meal is eaten with protein and carbohydrates, hunger will not hit for two or three hours, and fat will not be stored in the body.

Good sources of protein include egg whites, chicken or turkey breast, and buffalo. Complex carbohydrates include potatoes, pastas, sweet potatoes, rice, oatmeal, cream of wheat or rice, and vegetables. Simple carbohydrates include fruit, which elevates blood sugar quickly and releases insulin. When fruit is eaten, it is better to eat the fruit with a meal including appropriate protein and carbohydrates. However, fruit can be a snack.

In conclusion, always eat protein and carbohydrates together, so fat will not be stored in the body. DO NOT MISS MEALS! And by all means BE CONSISTENT!

30

6 How To Stay Thin Forever

Keeping weight down requires losing slowly and steadily, and most of all, being consistent with the eating right schedule and work-out program.

After changing eating choices, most of my clients lose approximately three to four pounds the first week of the exercise program. Then, a weight loss of approximately one pound per week can be expected.

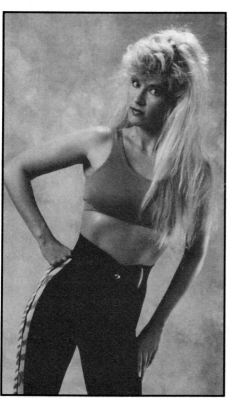

I like to do some sort of exercise each day, whether it is teaching a body-sculpting class, taking an aerobic class, or working with weights. Exercise is critical! Think this formula: Eating plus exercise equals energy.

Successful eaters DO cheat. Plan a cheat day! However, return to eating right the next day. Be warned! After cheating, the body rebels. No matter how wonderful the food tastes going down, once the body has adjusted to eating right with the proper balance of good, healthy, food, the shock of cheating, or eating fatty foods, will be difficult to tolerate.

If it is not cheat day, and the need for something forbidden is felt, treat yourself to something other than food. Instead of eating fattening food, purchase a new, exercise leotard to celebrate. Looking good and feeling good makes exercise more fun! Learn that it is okay to be spoiled. Find a special place to alleviate stress. Seek surroundings with peace and beauty. Take time to be pampered.

That is why I stress that part of food preparation is presentation. Make the food look even more deliciousby elaborate or whimsical table settings. Have a fun theme. Go Mexican or Italian with dinner decorations. Don't keep the silver for only special, holiday dinners. China and a fancy tablecloth really will make food taste more opulent.

Feel good about yourself! Feel good about food!

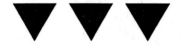

7 Tips For Eating Right

Eat! You must eat to lose weight. When you don't eat, your body immediately goes into a defensive mode and thinks, "I better store this food as fat, because I will need the energy later on." Eat high-volume, low-fat food, and you won't be hungry.

Don't count calories! Remember, if you're on a 1,000 calorie a day diet, those calories can all be consumed in the form of chocolate chip cookies, and you will feel terrible. Instead, be knowledgeable about fat content. Learn to think in grams. Balance and substitution are the keys to healthy eating habits.

Set Goals! Don't expect to lose weight immediately. Pounds didn't accumulate overnight, and they won't disappear overnight. Women who have gone through the eat-right program lose three to four pounds the first week and then continue to lose a pound per week, if exercise is included in the schedule. It takes time to change eating habits, so take one step at a time. For example, if you have never consistently eaten breakfast, then concentrate on eating right at breakfast. If soft drink addition is a downfall, start cutting down on the sodas as the second goal, and so on! Personalize your program.

Be a wise consumer! Learn to read labels carefully. Don't just read the front of the label. Be wise about content labeling. Fat and sodium content in foods can be particularly confusing. If the fat content is not labeled, don't buy it! Learn to look for hidden fat in food products. Lard is pure fat, and monosodium glutamate is sodium. New standards are being adopted by the FDA to guarantee food product labeling be accurate. Until these standards are used nationwide, learn to make healthy choices. For example, reduced calorie means that a product must have one-third fewer calories than the regular product. Low-fat means that a product must have one-third less fat than the traditional product. In other words, if the product has reduced or less fat than the original product, the amount of reduction may still not be appropriate for substitution choices. One slice of cheese that is normally fourteen grams of fat can be "reduced" to seven grams of fat, but so what! That is still too much fat to consume at one meal. Fat is in food. One boneless, skinless chicken breast, with absolutely nothing on it, still has six grams of fat. A plain, baked potato without toppings of any sort still has two to three grams of fat. The point is, the fat is there. Acknowledge the fat content of food. The fat content of food is hidden only to the unknowing consumer.

Exercise! It's true...exercise is a must. Find an activity you enjoy, and not dread, and do it! You'll be amazed how well you feel, how well you sleep, how well you look! Your energy level will increase with exercise. Your attitude will change with the eat-right program. You will lose weight! Enjoyment in exercise can be found at the gym, the Y, a church, a school, your backyard, down your street, around your block, on television, by tape. You can exercise with a group or alone. Just do it! And make sure that if you travel to exercise, don't drive over a few miles. If you have to go too far to get to the place where you plan to exercise, you are more likely to skip lessons or abandon the program. Your local gym is a wonderful place to exercise, make friends, get personalized training, and lose weight.

Grill! Invest in a gas grill for the home. All surface fat drains out of chicken, meat, and fish when grilled. Grilling adds wonderful flavor to meat quickly. If meats aren't grilled, broiling or microwaving, with added seasonings, will suffice for low-fat cooking.

Spray, don't grease! Use vegetable spray to coat all cooking utensils to guard against sticking. Use the spray to saute vegetables or make egg omelets. Spray directly on meat to aid cooking. These sprays now come in olive oil and butter flavorings.

Steam or microwave! Always steam or microwave vegetables. Take the foil or outer wrapping off a box of frozen vegetables, and place the box in the microwave. Perfectly steamed vegetables will be ready in five minutes without any mess or dirty dishes!

Don't serve meals family style but serve all of the family the same meal! Stop serving meals family style at the dinner table. When all of the food is displayed, it is too easy to overeat. Seconds are forbidden. Don't make one meal for the family then single yourself out, as a dieter, by having to cook something else for yourself, or even worse, having to eat a prepared diet meal or by only having something liquid. The whole family will benefit

34

from low-fat cooking and eating. Children will learn to eat wonderful, low-fat meals and set a pattern for the rest of their lives.

Don't skip meals! Simply, make and take the time to eat. Eat three, planned meals daily. Remember, you must eat to lose weight, but you must eat right. With this program, fast food eating is allowed as long as the proper menu items are ordered. Grilled chicken sandwiches on whole wheat bread or bun and plain baked potatoes are featured on most fast food menus today. Cheating is allowed if planned for and all on the same day. Low-fat substitution can be learned and favorite recipes can be prepared.

Stay away from soft drinks, regular or diet! Regular soft drinks have a high sugar and calorie count and often contain too much caffeine. Diet drinks are high in sodium content and are sweetened with one of two artificial sweeteners. Sodium causes water retention. Simply, not enough data is available to date on the long range effects of artificial sweeteners. If sugar is needed, use sugar, but use it sparingly. At least, the way in which the body assimilates sugar has long been understood. Drink water!

Learn to special order! Dining out at a favorite restaurant is allowed on the eating right program; however, learn to special order. Take advantage of the chef's creativity. Request low-fat food preparation and substitution. Ask for the sauces and dressings to be served on the side. If enough people request these foods, changes will be made to make low-fat food preparation more available.

Learn smart food/vitamin/mineral combinations! The maximum benefit of important vitamin and minerals can be released when food combinations are balanced. For example, drinking orange juice with a whole-grain cereal helps the iron in the cereal to increase the benefits of the Vitamin C in the juice. Plums and strawberries emulsify fat. Just as appropriate vitamin and mineral combinations can be enhanced by taking them with certain foods, vitamin and minerals can cancel each other out. Don't take calcium supplements and drink soft drinks. The phosphorous in soft drinks will block the absorption of calcium. The supplement is wasted.

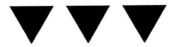

8 Grocery Shopping List

Good eating habits begin with a trip to the grocery store. Have items on hand to make low-fat cooking easy and quick. This list will help with the initial, reorganization of your kitchen. If these items are staples in the home, high-fat substitution and reversion will be avoided. The list was compiled from the recipes which follow. However, learn to experiment with family recipes and old favorites. Be creative! Substitute! You have everything to lose!

chicken and turkey, skinless and
  boneless
fish, shrimp, crab
veal
buffalo

eggs for egg whites
buttermilk
skim milk
non-fat yogurt
Romano cheese
Parmesan cheese
non-fat cheddar cheese
non-fat mozarella cheese
Neufatchel cheese

rice and rice mixes
couscous
pasta

cream of wheat
oats and oatmeal
oat flour
whole wheat flour

Dijon mustard
regular mustard
hot pepper sauce
non-fat mayonnaise or,
non-fat Miracle Whip
non-fat salad dressings
picante sauce
low-sodium soy and,
low-sodium teriyaki sauce
Worchestershire sauce
light syrup (maple)
molasses
honey
ketchup
red wine vinegar
balsamic vinegar

corn starch
baking powder, baking soda
vegetable spray in asstd.
  colors
lemon juice
anchovy paste
olive oil

American Heart Assn. Herbs
Molly McButter flavorings
basil
cayenne pepper
powdered mustard
thyme
cilantro
garlic cloves
oregano
Italian seasonings
onion powder
paprika
poultry seasoning
minced parsley
fines herbs
fresh dill
cardoman
rosemary
vanilla extract

"Simply Potatoes" (in frozen foods)
frozen, unsweetened fruits
frozen, microwave vegetables

spreadable fruit (don't call it jelly)
raisins

pizza crust
French bread
bread crumbs
ready-made crepes (in dairy case)
Guiltless Chips (in Mex. food section)
low-sodium chicken broth

potatoes (red, baking, and sweet)
Italian tomatoes
scallions
celery
bell peppers, green and red
bananas
apples

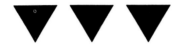

9 Exercise, Weight Training, & Aerobics

I don't weigh or measure my clients before starting the eating and right and exercise program with them. It is too easy to let the scale dictate how well you feel, how good you think you look, and how you feel about yourself. When the scale doesn't indicate immediate results, it's too easy to become discouraged and abandon the program. The weight loss will not come quickly, just steadily and gradually.

When we were young, our bodies burned calories and fat just by being alive. However, as we age, we burn fewer calories and store more fat. The bottom line is that exercising at least three or four days per week is necessary to change lifestyles and become fit and lean.

Weight training will add more muscle mass to the body while creating a new shape. This additional muscle mass will add more scale weight, even though you will be leaner. The body proportions will change, and indicators given on typical weight charts will be inaccurate and misleading for your body type. To build endurance first with a beginning weight training program, I suggest using light weights with high repetition.

Aerobic exercise will reduce body fat and the risk of heart disease, if the body temperature is raised for at least 30 to 40 minutes during each workout session. Begin slowly, and gradually work up to the optimum exercise level. This can be easily achieved by a difference in the music used during the exercise period. The basic program I developed for the eat right, don't diet program begins with a lecture session about general nutrition. The next four sessions are held in the gym to begin working out properly.

The first workout is a leg routine, which should be done twice a week, to concentrate on hips, thighs, and buttocks. The second workout is for back, biceps, and calves. The third workout concentrates on chest, shoulders, and triceps. Abdominal muscles should be worked after each session to build strength. Each workout ends with a personal choice, forty minute aerobic activity.

Doing aerobics at least four days a week helps keep my

weight down and my endurance at peak levels. I encourage all of my clients to do the same. I usually start them with a ten minute session on an inclined treadmill. We gradually build up to 40 minutes after each weight workout.

MONDAY:

Back and Hamstrings:

(three exercises for each muscle group)

Back:

    Lat pulldown--warm-up with three plates--20 repetitions
    Rowing
    Seated Row

Hamstrings:

    Leg curl
    Straight leg deadlifts
    Inverted leg press or squats
    Abdominal exercises

Then for pure enjoyment, I will take or teach an aerobic class.

TUESDAY:

Take or teach a body sculpting class and do repetition with light weights.

WEDNESDAY:

Chest and Biceps:

Chest:

    Bench press--warm-up with the bar for 15 repetitions
    Cable cross-overs
    Flys

Biceps:

    Alternating bicep curls
    Hammers
    Bicep curl machine

THURSDAY:

Take or teach body sculpting class choreographed to music.

FRIDAY:

Shoulders and Triceps:

Shoulders:

    Shoulder press
    Pitcher pours with free weights
    Rear deltoid machine
    Abdominal exercises
    Aerobics for at least 50 minutes

SATURDAY:

Easy Leg Day

    Leg press--warm-up with 20 repetitions
    Leg extensions
    Rotary hip machine
    Hyperextensions with 30 pound plate held to chest
    Aerobics

SUNDAY: REST!

The preceding is a typical weight training and aerobic workout for my week. I am not recommending that this is where you should begin; however, it could help set your goals. This schedule is changed periodically to relieve boredom and to challenge different muscle groups in my body. At times, I change the time of day of workouts to shock my system in a good way. This workout was developed for gym training and uses many high-tech machines.

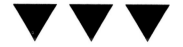

PART II

PART II

Table of Contents

Breakfast Recipes

I have always eaten and enjoyed breakfast. Eating breakfast will help keep weight down and energy levels up. Make time for breakfast!

By changing some old habits and by experimenting with new recipes, you can start the day off right with these breakfast entrees.

Don't forget to take vitamin and mineral supplements at breakfast time to maximize the benefits. Iron and calcium are especially needed at the beginning of a new day.

Crustless Quiche

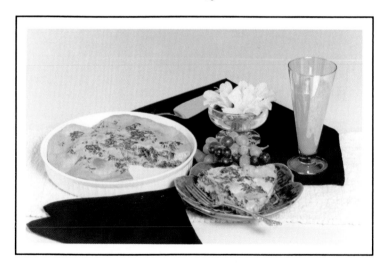

Breakfast Recipes

Crustless Quiche

In traditional quiche recipes, fat is found in the crust and the egg yokes. By eliminating the crust and using only egg whites, I created a high-protein, low-fat entree to be served at breakfast, lunch, or dinner. Serve with a small, side salad topped with non-fat dressing and crunchy, French bread.

1 package frozen, chopped spinach
1/2 cup scallions, chopped
1 teaspoon American Heart
    Association herbs
1 cup non-fat cheddar
    cheese, shredded

In a blender:
1 cup whole wheat flour
6 egg whites
1/2 cup skim milk
1 cup water
1-1/2 teaspoon mustard
1/4 cup non-fat mayonnaise

Remove foil wrapping, if any, from package of frozen spinach. Microwave spinach in the box for five minutes. Blend all ingredients together and pour into a quiche pan coated with vegetable spray. Bake at 400 degrees for 35 to 40 minutes. Remove from oven and let stand for five minutes before serving.

> 295 calories
> 3 grams fat
> 42 grams carbohydrates
> 12 grams protein
> Makes six to eight servings

Breakfast Recipes

Big Lou's Banana Pancakes

Lou Ferrigno, The Incredible Hulk from television fame, came to help celebrate the grand opening of the second World Gym in Houston in 1987. These pancakes are his favorite.

6 egg whites
2 cups oat bran flour
1 cup oats
2 bananas, ripe
1-1/2 cups water
1 teaspoon cinnamon
1 teaspoon cardamom

In large mixing bowl, mash bananas with a large spoon. Add remaining ingredients, and let stand for one of two minutes. Coat a large skillet with vegetable spray and turn on very high heat. Pour 1/3 cup of batter for each pancake. When edges are hard and bubbles are firm, turn each pancake and cook for one minute. Remove and serve with fresh slices of bananas.

210 calories for 3 pancakes
4 grams fat
12 grams protein
42 grams carbohydrates
Makes 12 pancakes

Gingerbread Waffle

These waffles are one of my favorite treats for Sunday morning or for entertaining breakfast guests. The smell is wonderful! It's ginger-bread without the fat and calories. Top with a favorite, fresh fruit or light syrup.

1-1/4 cups all-purpose flour
1 teaspoon baking powder
1 teaspoon baking soda
1 teaspoon ground ginger
1 teaspoon ground cinnamon
1/4 cup sugar
6 egg whites
1 cup buttermilk
1/2 cup molasses

Combine first six ingredients and set aside in large bowl. In another bowl, combine egg whites, buttermilk, and molasses and mix well. Add to flour mixture, and stir until well-blended. Bake in preheated waffle iron coated with vegetable spray.

150 calories per waffle
2 grams fat
32 grams carbohydrates
6 grams protein
Makes 6 large waffles or 12 small waffles

Breakfast Recipes

Apple Oatcakes

To spice up regular oatcakes, I added fresh apples to the batter. Serve with the egg white omelet recipe, and you will have a complete, lasting, nutritious breakfast.

6 egg whites
2 cups oat bran flour
1 cup oats
1-1/2 cups water
1 teaspoon cinnamon
1 teaspoon apple pie spice
3 apples, cored and chopped

In a large bowl, mix first six ingredients together. Add the apples, and let stand for 20 minutes. Coat a large skillet with vegetable spray and heat to high. Drop 1/3 cup of batter into skillet for each oatcake. Cook until edges are firm and batter has bubbled evenly. Turn and cook two minutes on other side. Remove and serve with applesauce or fresh apple slices.

195 calories
3 grams fat
32 grams carbohydrates
6 grams protein
Makes 12 pancakes

Breakfast Recipes

Breakfast Burritos

One large, flour tortilla has four grams of fat and 65 calories. Ready-made crepes (found in the dairy case) are a wonderful substitu-tion to make this Mexican favorite.

4 ready-made crepes
8 egg whites
1/2 green pepper, chopped
2 Italian tomatoes, chopped
2 scallions, chopped
1/2 cup mushrooms, chopped
1 8 ounce package non-fat cheddar cheese, shredded
picante sauce
vegetable spray

Coat a large skillet with vegetable spray and heat to high. Cook green pepper, scallions, and mushrooms for one minute. Add egg whites and scramble until cooked. Add chopped tomatoes and cheese. Place crepes on cookie sheet lightly coated with vegetable spray. Spoon egg white mixture down the middle of each crepe. Fold over crepe edges. Pour picante sauce down the middle of each crepe, and oven bake at 350 degrees for 10 minutes.

80 calories
1 gram fat
15 grams protein

10 grams carbohydrates
Makes four servings

Breakfast Recipes

Yogurt, Oats and Raisins by Keith Klein

Keith Klein is a top nutritionist who has helped many body builders achieve their goals and win championships. This recipe tastes great and makes eating right very easy. This recipe makes an excellent snack or breakfast food.

    8 ounces (1 container) plain, light yogurt
    1/3 cup raw oats
    2 tablespoons raisins

Mix all ingredients together and let stand in the refrigerator for at least 30 minutes before eating.

110 calories
2 grams fat
42 grams carbohydrates
3 grams protein
Makes one serving

51

Breakfast Recipes

Egg White Omelet

I make this omelet every morning for breakfast in a very short time. Add to your meal, a serving of cream of wheat flavored with cinnamon raisins and vanilla or one serving of breakfast potatoes (see recipe), and one piece of dry toast with spreadable fruit for an excellent, low-fat, high-energy breakfast.

> 1 scallion, chopped
> 1 Italian tomato, chopped or sliced
> 3 to 4 egg whites
> non-fat cheddar cheese, shredded
> bacon flavor seasoning (Molly McButter)
> vegetable spray

Coat a small skillet with vegetable spray and set on high heat. Add scallions and cook for one minute. Add egg whites and let cook, lifting edges with spatula to let uncooked egg slide to the bottom of pan. Add chopped tomatoes and cheese to one side and fold over egg. Sprinkle with flavored seasoning and remove to plate.

> 134 calories
> 1 gram fat
> 12 grams protein
> 6.6 grams carbohydrates
> Makes two servings

Breakfast Recipes

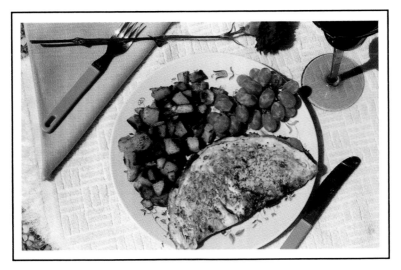

Egg White Omelet

Breakfast Recipes

Breakfast Potatoes

Simply Potatoes has come out with a bag of ready to cook, raw potatoes. These are shredded, fresh potatoes which come plain or with onion. They are quick and easy and are wonderful with the egg white omelet or as a side dish with lunch or dinner.

1 cup Simply Potatoes or 1 new, red potato, cut into squares
1/8 teaspoon salt substitute
1/2 teaspoon onion powder
pepper to taste
pinch of rosemary
pinch of thyme
vegetable spray

In small skillet coated with vegetable spray, cook potatoes, with all seasonings, on high heat. Lower heat setting and cover. Let cook several more minutes. Remove lid and stir until all sides of potatoes are browned. Remove and serve immediately.

95 calories
0.2 grams fat
22 grams carbohydrates
2 grams protein
Makes one serving

Breakfast Recipes

Raspberry French Toast

Raspberries are my favorite fruit; however, they are not always available fresh, so I keep raspberry spreadable fruit on hand in my refrigerator. If raspberries aren't your passion, choose another spreadable fruit flavor to make this wonderful, breakfast recipe.

2 tablespoons raspberry spreadable fruit
2 tablespoons Neufatchel cheese
8 slices of French bread
4 egg whites
1/4 cup skim milk
1 teaspoon honey
1/2 teaspoon vanilla extract
vegetable spray

Combine spreadable fruit and Neufatchel cheese and stir well. Spread evenly over four slices of French bread. Top with remaining slices of bread. Combine egg whites, skim milk, honey, and vanilla. Beat well with wire whisk. Carefully dip each sandwich into egg white mixture. Coat a large skillet with vegetable spray and set on high heat. Cook sandwiches for three minutes on each side. Remove and serve with fresh fruit. A sprinkle of powdered sugar is allowed.

262 calories
3.9 grams fat
10.7 grams protein
46 grams carbohydrates
Makes four servings

Appetizers, Soups and Salads

There is no reason why entertaining at home must be done with high-fat, high-calorie foods. These recipes will help serve guests pleasing appetizers, soups, and salads which are low in fat and low in calorie, without sacrificing taste or appearance.

Stuffed Mushrooms

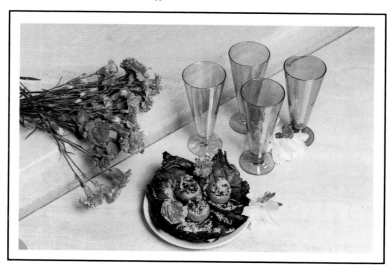

Stuffed Mushrooms

These are one of my favorite appetizers; however, the usual stuffed mushroom is high in fat. This delicious recipe reduces the fat in the stuffing significantly. So, enjoy!

24 large, fresh mushrooms
1 package frozen spinach, chopped
1 clove garlic, minced
2 scallions, chopped
1 8-ounce package Neufatchel cheese
1/2 cup bread crumbs
3/4 teaspoon dry mustard
1/4 teaspoon ground nutmeg
pepper to taste
2-1/2 tablespoons Parmesan cheese

Clean mushrooms. Remove and chop stems. Remove foil or outer wrappings from box of spinach and microwave for five minutes. Cook garlic for one minute in skillet coated with vegetable spray. Remove from heat. Spray mushroom caps and place in baking dish. Stir chopped mushroom stems and scallions into garlic. Cook until tender. Combine spinach, Neufatchel cheese, and next four ingredients in a medium bowl. If the Neufatchel cheese needs to be softened, microwave for 30 seconds in a small bowl. Add mushroom stem mixture and stir well. Spoon spinach mixture into mushroom caps and sprinkle with Parmesan cheese. Bake at 375 degrees for 15 minutes.

80 calories per mushroom
2 grams fat
3 grams protein
16 grams carbohydrates

Egg White Crepe Cups

These crepe cups make a fun and filling snack, or they can be served at brunch to satisfy friends and family with a new taste treat. Guests will never know this pretty dish is healthy for them because of the low fat content.

6 ready-made crepes
8 egg whites
2 scallions, chopped
1/2 cup non-fat cheddar cheese, shredded
2 fresh Italian tomatoes, chopped
1 teaspoon onion powder
vegetable spray
paprika

Spray muffin cups with vegetable spray and carefully place one crepe in each cup. Add chopped scallions, cheddar cheese, and tomatoes. Whip egg whites and onion powder together in a blender. Pour egg white mixture into each crepe, filling almost to the top. Sprinkle with paprika. Bake at 350 degrees for 35 to 40 minutes.

80 calories per crepe cup
1 gram fat
10 grams carbohydrates
18 grams protein
Makes six servings

Chili Con Queso with Guiltless Chips

Guiltless Chips are available in most grocery stores in the Mexican food section. These chips are baked rather than fried and have only a small amount of fat compared to the traditional version. No wonder they are called, guiltless!

1 8-ounce package non-fat cheddar cheese, shredded
1 small jar picante sauce
vegetable spray

Melt cheese in a saucepan coated with vegetable spray. Add picante sauce and stir constantly over low heat until blended.

50 calories per cup
0 grams fat
10 grams carbohydrates
3 grams protein

Appetizers, Soups, and Salads

Baked New Potatoes

When these potatoes are baked at a high temperature, they are crisp on the outside and moist and meaty on the inside. Serve an arrangement of non-fat condiments for potato toppings in small bowls. Allow two potatoes per person.

 8 potatoes
 8 ounces non-fat cheddar and mozzarella cheese, shredded
 chopped scallions
 plain, non-fat yogurt
 chopped parsley
 assorted flavors of Molly McButter seasonings

   Wash potatoes and pierce once with a fork. Place on wire rack in the oven for one hour at 450 degrees. When potatoes are done, keep warm in covered serving dish. Can be served with a favorite entree or as a low-fat appetizer.

95 calories per potato	2 grams protein
1 gram fat	Makes four servings
22 grams carbohydrates	

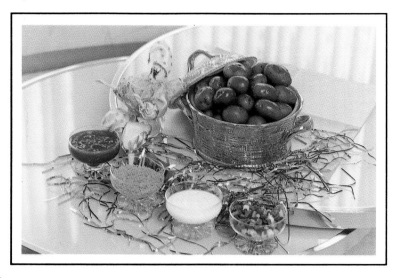

Appetizers, Soups, and Salads

Low-Fat Fresh Vegetable Dip

This dip is wonderful served with Guiltless Chips (found in the Mexican food section of most grocery stores). This low-fat appetizer can be prepared the day before a party to give additional time for other recipes.

1 10-ounce package frozen, chopped spinach
1 cup non-fat yogurt, plain
2 tablespoons lemon juice
1/2 cup fresh minced parsley
2 scallions, chopped
1/2 cup non-fat Miracle Whip or mayonnaise
1 teaspoon fines herbs
1 teaspoon minced, fresh dill
pepper to taste
paprika

With foil or wrapping removed, microwave spinach in its box. Remove and drain. Squeeze dry. Transfer spinach to mixing bowl and add remaining ingredients, except paprika. Mix well. Sprinkle with paprika, cover and refrigerate. Serve cold.

60 calories per cup
0.2 grams fat
22 grams carbohydrates
9 grams protein

61

Party Turkey Meatballs

These are an unusual appetizer, or they can be served as a main course meal. The taste is tangy, slightly sweet, and unique, with the addition of the grape flavor. The meatballs can be frozen, without the sauce, for a quick meal. For a main meal, serve with rice or pasta and a dinner salad.

2 pounds lean ground turkey
1/2 cup Simply Potatoes, shredded
2 egg whites
1 bottle chili sauce
4 tablespoons grape, spreadable fruit
1 teaspoon Worcestershire sauce
 pepper to taste

Combine first four ingredients in a large bowl and mix well. Season with pepper. Form meat mixture into balls and set aside. Blend chili sauce, Worcestershire sauce, and spreadable fruit in a large skillet on medium heat. Add meatballs and cover. Turn down heat to low and cook for 30 minutes. Stir occasionally. When ready to serve, transfer to a chafing dish or fondue pot. Pour sauce over meatballs and serve warm.

35 calories per meatball
1 gram fat
6 grams protein
0.6 grams carbohydrates
Makes 50 meatballs

Appetizers, Soups, and Salads

Low-Fat Spinach Balls

Party guests will love this appetizer and not realize how low in fat it is. Spinach balls can be partially baked for ten minutes at 350 degrees and then frozen. Thaw and bake for an additional 10 to 15 minutes. It's always nice to have something prepared in the freezer for a special treat on hurried nights.

    12 egg whites
    2 packages frozen spinach, chopped
    2 cups herb stuffing mix
    3 scallions, finely chopped
    1/2 cup Parmesan cheese
    1 teaspoon poultry seasoning
    pepper to taste

Beat egg whites in a large bowl. Add remaining ingredients and blend well. Roll into 1-1/2 inch sized balls. Transfer to a baking sheet. Bake for 20 minutes at 350 degrees.

    35 calories per spinach ball
    0.6 grams fat
    11 grams carbohydrates
    2 grams protein
    Makes six dozen

Appetizers, Soups, and Salads

Crab Cakes with Red Pepper Sauce

I had to develop a low-fat version of this classic appetizer, because it is one of my husband's favorites. The red pepper sauce may be served on the plate with the crab cakes in the center or served on the side.

1 pound lump, crab meat
1 shallot, peeled and finely chopped
1 tablespoon all-purpose flour
4 egg whites, lightly beaten
3 scallions, chopped
1 cup Italian bread crumbs
1 tablespoon fresh parsley, chopped
1 tablespoon fresh dill, chopped
vegetable spray
pepper to taste

Saute the shallot in a skillet coated with vegetable spray. In a large bowl, gently mix all ingredients together, including shallot. Coat the skillet again with vegetable spray and set on medium high heat. Form the crab meat mixture into small, thick pancakes, and cook in skillet for three to four minutes on each side. Serve immediately with red pepper sauce.

Red Pepper Sauce

4 red, bell peppers
1 large carton, non-fat yogurt, plain
salt (optional)

Grill red peppers or broil in oven until skin is black. Let cook and peel the black skin from peppers. Place the peppers in blender and add yogurt. Blend well. Pour into saucepan and heat.

102 calories
2 grams fat
12 grams carbohydrates

4 grams protein
Makes appetizers for six

64

Appetizers, Soups, and Salads

Couscous Soup

Couscous is a Moroccan pasta which can be found in the rice section of most grocery stores. As an ethnic food, couscous has been available for years in speciality stores. However, as the everyday consumer becomes aware of its qualities, it has become more widely available. Think of couscous as being half pasta, half rice. It cooks up fluffy like rice but has the texture of pasta.

2 cans low-sodium chicken broth (14-1/2 ounces each)
2 bay leaves
1 scallion, chopped
1-1/2 teaspoons ground cumin
1/2 cup couscous
1 tablespoon lemon juice

Simmer first five ingredients together in a large saucepan over medium heat for ten minutes. Add couscous and lemon juice and cover. Simmer for five more minutes, and this unusual soup is ready to serve!

180 calories
2 grams fat
28 grams carbohydrates
4 grams protein
Makes two to four servings

Potato-Broccoli Chowder

Since my childhood days in Michigan, potato-broccoli chowder has always been one of my favorites. This is a low-fat version of that Midwestern classic using skim milk instead of the traditional chowder cream.

2 packages frozen broccoli, chopped
4 medium potatoes, baked and cut into bite-sized squares
3 scallions, chopped
1 clove garlic, minced
4 quarts low-sodium chicken broth
1/4 cup skim milk
pepper to taste

Remove any foil or outer wrappings from boxes of broccoli and microwave both boxes for ten minutes. In large pot sprayed with vegetable spray, cook scallions and garlic for one minute. Add broccoli, potatoes, chicken broth, and skim milk. Bring to a boil and add pepper. Reduce heat and simmer an additional five minutes.

225 calories
3 grams fat
42 grams carbohydrates
12 grams protein
Serves eight to ten

Appetizers, Soups, and Salads

Chilled Cucumber Soup

Substituting non-fat yogurt for the heavy cream in this recipe is the low-fat secret. Rewrite your own favorites recipes using non-fat yogurt. There is a healthy difference in the fat content but not in taste.

1 large cucumber, chopped
1 small yellow onion, chopped
2 chicken bouillon cubes
1-1/2 cups non-fat yogurt, plain
1 tablespoon minced chives
fresh dill for garnish

Combine cucumber and onion in a medium saucepan. Add water just to cover. Stir in bouillon cubes and simmer until cucumber and onions are tender. Let cool, cover, and refrigerate. When ready to serve, blend in yogurt and chives. Spoon into serving bowls and garnish with fresh dill.

80 calories per bowl
0.2 grams fat
1.0 carbohydrates
trace of protein
Makes four servings

Healthy Gazpacho

This soup is a summertime favorite because it is served chilled. Try serving this low-fat version for a spicy treat anytime.

4 ripe tomatoes, peeled and diced
1 large cucumber, peeled and chopped
1 green pepper, chopped
1 medium onion, finely chopped
1 clove garlic, minced
1 cup low-sodium tomato juice or non-alcoholic Bloody Mary
mix 1/4 cup
non-fat Italian salad dressing

Mix together and chill for several hours in airtight container.
Serve cold!

54 calories
0.5 grams fat
11.5 carbohydrates
2.4 grams protein
Makes four servings

Appetizers, Soups, and Salads

Tortellini and Chicken Soup

Americans love to eat Italian, but most recipes for this type of ethnic food are packed with fat and calories from the cheeses, sauces, and pastas. Soup is a wonderful way to fill up without filling out on high-calorie foods. This version of a favorite, Italian soup cuts calorie intake almost in half by a difference in chicken preparation.

4-1/2 quarts low-sodium chicken broth
1 package tortellini noodles
1 pound boneless, skinless chicken breasts, cut in squares
1/2 pound mushrooms, sliced
1 red, bell pepper
1 cup cooked, brown rice
2 teaspoons tarragon leaves

In large pot, bring chicken broth to a boil. Add tortellini and cook four minutes. Add remaining ingredients and return to a boil. Reduce heat, cover, and simmer until chicken is done, about three minutes. Ladle into bowls and sprinkle with Parmesan cheese.

201 calories per serving
4 grams fat
21 grams carbohydrates
19 grams protein
Makes eight servings

Turkey-Rice Soup

Left-over turkey can be a problem after a holiday dinner. This soup solves that, as well as providing enough protein and carbohydrates to help maintain low-fat eating the rest of the season. Try it, too, for an all-year favorite using fresh turkey meat.

4-1/2 quarts low-sodium chicken broth
1 cup wild rice
2 cups cooked turkey meat
3 stalks celery, chopped thick
4 scallions, chopped
1 can low-sodium stewed tomatoes (14-1/2) ounces
1 tablespoon sage
1 tablespoon marjoram leaves
4 cloves garlic, minced
2 bay leaves
pepper to taste

Combine all ingredients in large pot and bring to a boil. Reduce heat and simmer about five minutes.

245 calories
5.3 grams fat
24 grams carbohydrates
26 grams protein
Makes eight to ten servings

Honey Mustard Dressing

Even though wonderful, non-fat salad dressings are now commercially available, it is still difficult to find a honey mustard dressing that doesn't contain egg yolks. Here is a recipe for a make at home, non-fat dressing to top a spinach salad. Garnish with non-fat, shredded mozzarella cheese and chopped egg whites for a real treat!

1 large carton non-fat yogurt, plain
1/2 cup mustard
3 tablespoons honey
1/4 cup red wine vinegar
dash of paprika
pepper to taste

12 calories per tablespoon
0.2 grams fat
25 grams carbohydrates
9 grams protein

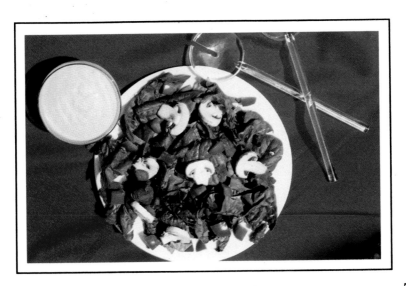

Appetizers, Soups, and Salads

Low-Fat Caesar Dressing

It's hard to believe a Caesar Salad low in fat can still taste wonderful! This salad is good for lunch or as a meal starter for guests at dinner.

1 large head Romaine lettuce, torn
1 cup sliced, fresh mushrooms
1/4 cup water
2 tablespoons grated Romano cheese
2 tablespoons red wine vinegar
1-1/2 teaspoons anchovy paste
1/2 teaspoon olive oil
2 cloves garlic
pepper to taste

Wash lettuce and mushrooms, and toss together in large bowl. In a blender, process the remaining ingredients, and pour over salad.

37 calories per 1 cup serving
1.4 grams of fat
3.9 grams carbohydrates
2.6 grams protein
Makes four to six servings

Appetizers, Soups, and Salads

Low-Calorie Coleslaw

Cabbage, broccoli, and cauliflower are high-fiber vegetables which should be eaten as often as possible. This coleslaw offers a tasty, low-calorie version of the traditional recipe, without the fat. Serve this as a change of pace dish instead of salad or steamed vegetables.

1 large cabbage
2 scallions, chopped fine
2 tablespoons lemon juice
3/4 cup non-fat mayonnaise or Miracle Whip
1 tablespoon caraway seeds
paprika
pepper to taste

Shred cabbage in a food processor. Add onion, lemon juice, and pepper. Stir in mayonnaise or dressing and caraway seeds. Chill before serving. Sprinkle with paprika.

30 calories per cup
0.2 grams fat
5.0 grams carbohydrates
1 gram protein
Makes six to eight servings

Low-Fat, Low-Calorie Main Dishes

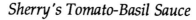

Eating three carrot sticks and one plain, boneless, skinless chicken breast is not my idea of a healthy dinner.

This is starvation! Low-fat cooking can be convenient and filling. There are easy ways to substitute or eliminate fat from most recipes if the ingredients are available in your kitchen for quick preparation. Main dishes should taste wonderful, be easy to prepare, and be low in fat. Once low-fat substitution is understood, try rewriting your favorite family recipes! It's fun and so good for you!

Sherry's Tomato-Basil Sauce

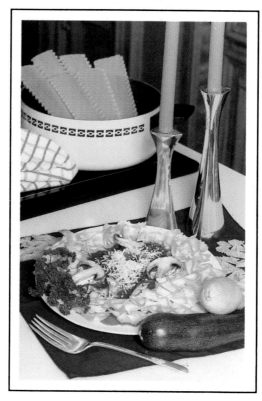

Sherry's Tomato-Basil Sauce

Make this great sauce in large quantities to have on hand in the refrigerator. Pour over favorite pasta dishes or use in a low-fat pizza. This sauce is used in the Turkey-Spinach Lasagne (see recipe). Sauce will keep in the refrigerator for four or five days and can be frozen in small bags for use in a number of different recipes. Experiment with this non-traditional, Italian sauce yourself!

> 2 large cartons of Pomi tomato sauce with tomato chunks
> 4 cloves garlic, minced
> 4 teaspoons oregano
> 4 teaspoons Italian seasoning
> 4 teaspoon basil. If fresh basil is available, chop 1 small
>   bunch.
> 1 cup red wine (optional)

Mix together all ingredients in large pot and bring to a boil. Reduce heat and simmer for five minutes. Remove from heat and let cool before placing in large air-tight container.

45 calories
0 grams fat
2 grams protein
10 grams carbohydrates
Makes six to eight servings

Pizza Crust

Americans eat 11 billion slices of pizza each year even though pizza is one of the most fattening foods on the market today. However, pizza does not have to be full of fat to be full of flavor. Instead of using pepperoni, sausage, and high-fat cheeses, substitute grilled chicken, turkey, or buffalo, and non-fat cheeses. Use chopped, fresh vegetables for extra toppings. The whole wheat crust recipe is even tastier than the traditional dough used for pizza. Pizza can still be on the menu, and made this new, healthier way, fat and calories will be cut drastically.

1-1/4 cups warm water
1 tablespoon honey
1 envelope dry yeast
1-1/2 cups all-purpose flour
2 cups whole wheat flour
olive oil vegetable spray

In a small bowl, combine warm water and honey. Sprinkle the yeast over the water, and stir until it dissolves, about one minute. In a large bowl, combine flours. Make a hole in the center of the flour mixture and add the yeast mixture. Use a wooden spoon to mix well until a soft dough forms. Turn dough onto a floured surface and form a dome, then flatten with floured hands. Fold like a business litter and form another dome. Place in a bowl sprayed with olive oil vegetable spray. This prevents dough from sticking or getting hard. Cover tightly, and set to rise in a warm place until it doubles in size, about 45 minutes. Roll out to desired thickness and shape to pizza pan. Bake at 500 degrees for ten minutes.

Topping:

Top crust with Tomato-Basil Sauce (see recipe) and other favorite toppings. Sprinkle with non-fat mozzarella and Parmesan cheese. Bake at 450 degrees for 15 minutes.

80 calories per slice of crust
3 grams fat
3 gram protein
26 grams carbohydrates
Makes eight slices

Low-Fat, Low-Calorie Main Dishes

Margherita Pizza

This low-fat version of a favorite, Italian pizza was created in honor of Italy's nineteenth century Queen Margherita.

pizza crust (see recipe)
olive oil vegetable spray
8 ounces non-fat mozzarella cheese, shredded
3 Italian tomatoes, sliced
2 tablespoons fresh oregano, chopped
3 tablespoons fresh basil, chopped
1/4 cup Parmesan cheese, shredded

Spread prepared pizza crust onto pizza pan. Spray crust with olive oil vegetable spray. Cover with non-fat mozzarella cheese. Arrange tomato slices over cheese and sprinkle with fresh oregano and Parmesan. Spray again with olive oil spray. Bake at 500 degrees for ten minutes. Remove and add chopped basil.

180 calories per slice
4 grams fat
38 grams carbohydrates
12 grams protein
Makes eight slices

Vegetarian Pizza

Chopped chicken, turkey, or buffalo may be added to this pizza for a quick, satisfying, low-fat, complete meal!

Choice of ingredients:

fresh broccoli	chopped spinach
asparagus	Italian tomatoes
yellow squash	carrots
zucchini	red or yellow peppers
green or red onions	

Choose at least two or three vegetables for best taste. Microwave chosen vegetables for two minutes to blanch and bring out natural, vibrant colors. Spray prepared pizza dough (see recipe) with olive oil vegetable spray. Spread crust with Tomato-Basil Sauce (see recipe) and top with non-fat mozzarella cheese. Arrange vegetables on sauce, and sprinkle with chopped garlic (two tablespoons) and one chopped scallion. Spray with olive oil spray. Bake at 500 degrees for eight to ten minutes.

95 calories per slice
3 grams fat
41 grams carbohydrates
4 grams protein
Makes eight slices

Low-Fat, Low-Calorie Main Dishes

Seafood Pizza

Any seafood lover will enjoy this quick and easy pizza, because the seafood cooks right on top of the pizza crust.

Tomato-Basil Sauce (see recipe)
pizza crust (see recipe)
2 tablespoons garlic, chopped
1 teaspoon lemon peel
3 tablespoons Parmesan cheese
Choice of fresh, cleaned shrimp, scallops, squid, or crab.

Spread pizza crust with Tomato-Basil Sauce and arrange raw seafood over sauce. Sprinkle with garlic, lemon, and Parmesan cheese. Spray vegetable spray over all ingredients. Spraying the pizza with vegetable spray helps cook the seafood while still keeping it moist. Bake for ten minutes at 500 degrees.

225 calories per slice
5 grams fat
39 grams protein
32 grams carbohydrates
Makes eight slices

Glazed Onion Pizza with Buffalo

Glazed onions and garlic give wonderful and unusual flavor to this hearty, but low-fat pizza. Serve with a side salad topped with non-fat salad dressing.

1 pound buffalo, grilled and chopped
3 onions, sliced and separated into rings
6 tablespoons garlic, minced
3 tablespoons thyme
1 bay leaf, crushed
pepper to taste
vegetable spray

Spray a large skillet generously with vegetable spray. Cook all ingredients on medium high heat for thirty minutes, until onions become caramelized. Stir frequently to scrape onions off the bottom of skillet. Spread mixture over whole wheat pizza crust (see recipe) and top with buffalo meat. Bake for ten minutes at 500 degrees. Grilled chicken or turkey can be substituted for the buffalo, and sliced Italian tomatoes, bell peppers, or zucchini can be added.

180 calories per slice
4 grams fat
10 grams protein
38 grams carbohydrates
Makes eight slices

Low-Fat, Low-Calorie Main Dishes

Turkey-Spinach Lasagne

I developed this recipe for Lasagne Lovers everywhere, and it is the house specialty in the Sports Cafe at World Gym. Serve with a salad topped with a non-fat, salad dressing and grilled, garlic bread.

8 turkey fillets, grilled or broiled
2 packages frozen spinach, chopped
4 cloves garlic, minced
1 onion, chopped
3 egg whites
1/4 cup Parmesan cheese
Tomato-Basil Sauce (see recipe)
1 large package lasagne noodles
8 ounces non-fat mozzarella cheese, shredded
vegetable spray

Spray a large, stew pot with vegetable spray. Cook onion and garlic together for one minute. Remove foil and outer wrappings from boxes of spinach and microwave on high for ten minutes. Add to ingredients in pot and stir. Add cooked turkey, egg whites, and Parmesan cheese. Mix thoroughly. Cook lasagne noodles according to package directions. Remove from water and drain. Spread bottom of large baking pan with tomato-basil sauce to cover generously. Add lasagne noodles to form one layer. Spoon turkey mixture over noodles and sprinkle with non- fat mozzarella cheese. Repeat layering until all ingredients have been used. Finish with a layer of noodles, tomato sauce, and cheese. Sprinkle with Parmesan cheese. Bake 40 minutes at 375 degrees. Remove from oven, and let stand for ten minutes before slicing.

550 calories
8 grams fat per serving
45 grams carbohydrates
32 grams protein
Makes eight to ten servings

81

Turkey Pasta Bake

This dish is really easy to prepare at home using frozen turkey meat leftover from the holidays, or use packaged frozen turkey from the grocer's freezer.

1 package frozen turkey meat, cut into chunks
2 cups Tomato-Basil Sauce (see recipe)
1 package pasta, use wide noodles with no egg yolks
8 ounces non-fat mozzarella cheese, shredded
Parmesan cheese

Cook pasta according to package directions. Drain and pour into large mixing bowl. Add turkey, sauce, and mix well. Pour into baking pan and sprinkle mozzarella cheese on top. Top with Parmesan cheese. Bake at 350 degrees for 40-45 minutes until golden brown on top.

325 calories
5 grams fat
31 grams carbohydrates
28 grams protein
Makes eight to ten servings

Low-Fat, Low-Calorie Main Dishes

Maple-Mustard Chicken

This chicken dish has a wonderfully unique flavor and lends itself well to being a holiday speciality. The aroma alone is delicious! Instead of using maple syrup, with the extra calories and sugar, substitute maple extract to achieve the unusual flavor. The extra sauce can be poured over pasta or baked potato. Acorn squash complements this entree well.

4 chicken breasts, boneless and skinless
2 capfuls maple extract
2 cans low-sodium chicken broth
4 tablespoons Dijon mustard
1 teaspoon dried thyme
pepper to taste

Coat chicken breasts with vegetable spray and grill three to four minutes on each side. Remove and keep warm. If a gas grill is unavailable, use the broiler pan in the oven. In large skillet, add chicken broth, maple extract, mustard, and thyme. Stir constantly until mixture boils. Reduce heat and simmer for 15 to 20 minutes. Pour sauce over chicken and serve.

194 calories
3.2 grams fat
24 grams protein
11 grams carbohydrates
Makes four servings

Cranberry Chicken

This recipe is another dish that can be a special holiday treat because of the cranberry sauce, or it can be served anytime for a no-fuss, main meal. Serve with rice or baked potato.

4 chicken breasts, skinless and boneless
1 16-ounce can of cranberry sauce
1 bottle non-fat French salad dressing
1 envelope onion soup mix

Combine all ingredients and marinate overnight. Arrange chicken pieces in baking dish and bake at 400 degrees for ten minutes. Serve immediately.

289 calories per chicken breast
6 grams fat
22 gram protein
20 grams carbohydrates
Makes four servings

Apricot-Mustard Chicken

This quick recipe adds wonderful and rather exotic flavors to everyday chicken. This chicken dish is featured once a week in the Sports Cafe of our World Gyms, and members realize they can eat low-fat and healthy without sacrificing taste.

4 chicken breasts, boneless and skinless
1 jar apricot nectar
3 tablespoons Dijon mustard
2 scallions, sliced lengthwise into narrow strips
vegetable spray

Pour apricot nectar and mustard into large pan coated with vegetable spray. Stir constantly until mustard dissolves and is boiling. Add chicken breasts and cook four minutes on each side. Cover and reduce heat. Cook for five more minutes. Place cooked chicken on a serving platter and pour sauce over meat. Garnish with scallions.

192 calories
3.2 grams fat
24 grams protein
9 grams carbohydrates
Makes four servings

Quick Sauteed Vegetables

The whole family will love vegetables sauteed in a teriyaki and vinegar sauce. Experiment with any fresh vegetable!

1 zucchini, cut into chunks or sliced
1 yellow squash, cut into chunks or sliced
1 scallion, chopped
1/4 cup red wine vinegar or balsamic vinegar
1 tablespoon light teriyaki sauce

In a small skillet, heat vinegar and teriyaki sauce. Bring to a boil. Add all vegetables and continue to cook until vegetables are done and coated with sauce mixture.

35 calories per serving
trace of fat
8 grams carbohydrates
1 gram protein
Makes one to two servings

Chicken Piquant

This recipe makes one of those party perfect dishes that is easy, yet elegant. The sauce can be made in the morning and left in the blender all day, if necessary.

6 chicken breasts, boneless and skinless
3/4 cups rose wine
1/2 cup reduced sodium soy sauce
1/2 cup low-sodium chicken broth
2 tablespoons water
1 clove garlic, sliced
1 teaspoon ground ginger
1/2 teaspoon oregano
1 tablespoon brown sugar

Mix all ingredients (except chicken) together in a blender. Allow to stand for at least one hour before preparation begins. Arrange chicken in baking dish. Pour sauce over chicken, cover tightly, and bake for 45 minutes at 350 degrees. Serve with wild rice and a steamed vegetable.

225 calories
6 grams fat
24 grams protein
11 grams carbohydrates
Makes six servings

Chicken in Raspberry Sauce

Use fresh raspberries, when in season, or substitute frozen, unsweetened raspberries to make this very different, chicken recipe. A drop of raspberry liqueur will add extra flavor to the sauce.

4 chicken breasts, boneless and skinless
1/4 teaspoon pepper
1/4 teaspoon garlic powder
1 10-ounce package frozen, whole unsweetened
    raspberries, thawed
1/4 cup water
1 tablespoon sugar
1 teaspoon raspberry liqueur, optional
vegetable spray

Combine pepper and garlic powder in a bowl and coat chicken breasts on both sides. Heat a large skillet, coated with vegetable spray, to medium high heat. Cook chicken two to three minutes on each side. Remove and keep warm. The raspberries may be pressed through a strainer to remove the seeds. Let the juice fall into the skillet. Add water, sugar, lemon peel, and liqueur. Bring to a boil, reduce heat, and let simmer. Place chicken back into skillet and cook for ten more minutes.

210 calories
4 grams fat
11 grams carbohydrates
24 grams protein
Makes four servings

Spinach-Chicken Stuffed Bread

Stuffed breads make a tasty treat for a buffet table. Serve your family this fun and filling meal, which comes complete with vegetables, protein, and carbohydrates. No one will be able to resist the aroma while the bread is baking. This recipe is very quick and easy to prepare, if most of the ingredients are stocked in your freezer.

1 package frozen bread dough containing two loaves; let thaw
1 package frozen chopped spinach; microwave in its box for five minutes, foil and outer wrappings removed
1 package frozen chopped, cooked chicken
2 scallions, chopped
1 cup sliced mushrooms
8 ounces non-fat mozzarella cheese, shredded
1 tablespoon Parmesan cheese
pepper to taste

Place bread dough on floured surface and mold into dome with floured hands. Flour rolling pin and roll out to one inch thickness. Sprinkle cooked spinach, onion, cooked chicken, mushrooms, mozzarella, Parmesan, and pepper onto bread dough in the above order. The dough may be folded several different ways. Folded widthwise, the dough will bake into a round ball. Folded into a circle, the dough will bake into a wreath. Folded lengthwise, the dough will bake into a long strip. Bake at 375 degrees for 30 minutes. Let stand for five minutes before slicing.

250 calories
4 grams fat
11 grams carbohydrates
24 grams protein
Makes eight servings

Sherry Veal Chops with Apples

The apples, sherry, cinnamon, and brown sugar add an unusual taste to these chops. Serve veal with Twice-Baked Potatoes (see recipe) and salad.

6 veal chops
3 large apples, sliced
1/2 cup dry sherry wine
1 teaspoon ground cinnamon
1/4 cup brown sugar
vegetable spray

In large skillet coated with vegetable spray, brown veal chops on both sides. Arrange apple slices on the bottom of a large, baking pan coated with vegetable spray. Sprinkle with cinnamon and brown sugar. Place veal chops over apples and pour sherry over all ingredients. Cover tightly and bake at 375 degrees for 1-1/2 to 2 hours.

250 calories
4.8 grams fat
22 grams protein
11 grams carbohydrates

90

Danny's Turkey Scallopini with Balsamic Vinegar

Balsamic vinegar adds so much flavor to this dish with very few calories. Other flavored vinegars or lemon juice may be substituted for balsamic vinegar. Use lean, turkey fillets for a good source of protein with only three grams of fat per serving. This is my husband's favorite dish for dinner!

8 turkey fillets
3/4 cup whole wheat flour seasoned with pepper
1/4 cup balsamic vinegar
1/2 cup low-sodium chicken broth
1-1/2 tablespoons low-sodium tomato paste

Lightly dust turkey fillets with whole wheat flour. In a large skillet coated with vegetable spray, cook turkey fillets on high heat until golden brown on both sides, about two minutes on each side. Remove and keep warm. Add vinegar, chicken broth, and tomato paste to skillet and bring to a boil. Return turkey fillets to skillet and simmer for five minutes. Remove turkey fillets to shallow serving dish and pour remaining sauce over fillets.

220 calories
3 grams fat
11 gram carbohydrates
22 grams protein
Makes four servings

Cinnamon-Lemon Turkey

This dish can be made quickly if most of the ingredients are kept as staples in the kitchen. Serve over bow tie pasta for a special treat.

> 2 boneless, skinless turkey breasts, cut into squares
> 3 scallions, chopped
> 2-1/2 cups low-sodium chicken broth
> 1 tablespoon garlic, minced
> 1 16-ounce can low-sodium tomatoes, drained and chopped
> 3 tablespoons low-sodium tomato paste
> 2 cinnamon sticks, broken in half
> 2 lemons
> 1-1/2 teaspoon oregano
> 1/8 teaspoon ground allspice
> whole wheat flour
> vegetable spray
> pepper to taste

Coat turkey pieces in whole wheat flour. In a large skillet coated with vegetable spray, cook turkey until lightly browned. Remove and set aside. In a saucepan coated with vegetable spray, cook onion until browned. Add garlic and cook for 30 seconds. Reduce heat and stir in tomatoes, tomato paste, cinnamon sticks, oregano, allspice, and lemon juice, pulp, and skins. Simmer for five minutes. Add chicken broth and turkey. Simmer for at least 30 minutes. Remove cinnamon sticks and lemon skins. Serve over pasta.

120 calories per serving
3 grams fat
11 gram carbohydrates
23 grams protein
Makes two servings

Turkey-Apple Sausage

Tasty, low-fat turkey sausage is still difficult to find at the grocery store. This turkey sausage recipe can be made at home quickly with guaranteed low-fat, great flavor.

1 pound lean, ground turkey
2 egg whites, beaten
1/2 cup bread crumbs
1/2 cup finely chopped apple
1 teaspoon ground sage
pepper to taste
(1 teaspoon cinnamon and 1 teaspoon ginger can be
    substituted for the sage and pepper, if desired)

In a medium bowl, combine egg whites, bread crumbs, apple, sage, and pepper. Add ground turkey and mix well. Shape into patties and cook on the broiler pan in the oven. These patties may also be open-flame grilled for four to five minutes on each side. Serve with egg whites in the morning or with rice for dinner!

73 calories
1 gram fat
14 grams protein
3 grams carbohydrates

Buffalo Chili

Chili is always a popular, hearty meal during the winter months. Making chili with buffalo meat instead of regular ground meat cuts the fat in this favorite recipe in half. Remember, buffalo has 50 per cent more protein and 40 per cent less fat than ground meat.

2 pounds ground buffalo
1 can chopped, low-sodium tomatoes, undrained
2 scallions, chopped
1 16-ounce can chili beans
1 16-ounce can kidney beans, optional
1/2 cup ketchup
1 teaspoon chili powder
1 teaspoon cayenne pepper
1 teaspoon garlic, minced
2 teaspoons cilantro
1 teaspoon thyme
1/2 teaspoon powdered mustard
ground pepper to taste

If possible, grill buffalo, or cook in skillet over medium, high heat until brown. In large pot, add all ingredients and bring to a boil. Reduce heat and simmer for 20 minutes. Serve hot!

150 calories per serving
3 grams fat
28 grams protein
32 grams carbohydrates
Makes ten to twelve servings

Turkey Burritos

This Mexican favorite makes a filling, tasty, and quick lunch or dinner dish. To get the South of the Border flavor without all the fat and calories, ready-made crepes (in the dairy case) are used instead of the traditional, flour tortillas made with lard.

1 package ground turkey meat (use only ground white
    turkey meat with no skin or dark meat included)
1 package (8) ready-made crepes
1 green pepper, chopped
1 small onion, chopped
2 small tomatoes, chopped
8 ounces non-fat cheddar cheese, shredded
picante sauce

Brown turkey meat in large skillet. Add green peppers and onions and cook for two to three minutes. Add chopped tomato. Place one crepe on cookie sheet and fill with turkey mixture lengthwise, then fold over edges of crepes. Repeat until all ingredients and all crepes are used. After folding, sprinkle with cheese down the middle of each crepe and top with picante sauce. Bake at 350 degrees for ten minutes.

225 calories per burrito
4.5 grams fat
23 grams protein
12 grams carbohydrates
Makes four servings

Chicken Fajitas

Ready-made crepes may be substituted for the flour tortillas to keep the fat and calories to a minimum in this Mexican recipe. Forget the avocado in any Mexican dish. Avocados have 280 calories and 30 grams of fat...each!

4 boneless, skinless chicken breasts, cut into strips
8 ready-made crepes
1 onion, chopped
1 red, bell pepper, sliced
1/4 teaspoon ground cumin
1/4 teaspoon paprika
1/4 teaspoon cayenne pepper
1/4 teaspoon garlic powder
1/4 teaspoon oregano
1/4 teaspoon thyme
1/2 cup low-sodium chicken broth
1 large tomato, chopped
8 ounces non-fat cheddar cheese, shredded
vegetable spray

In large skillet coated with vegetable spray, cook onion and pepper for five minutes on medium-high heat. Add all spices and chicken broth, and bring to a boil. Add chicken and cook for five more minutes. Spoon chicken into ready-made crepes. Roll up and fold edges over. Serve with picante sauce and non-fat condiments.

225 calories per fajita
3.2 grams fat
11 grams carbohydrates
24 grams protein
Makes four servings

Chicken Quesadillas

Quesadillas served in most Mexican restaurants are high in both fat and calories. This tasty version substitutes baked, ready-made crepes for the usual, fried flour tortillas.

4 boneless, skinless chicken breasts, grilled and cut into
strips
6 ready-made crepes
1 cup non-fat mozzarella cheese, shredded
6 tablespoons diced chili peppers
1 tomato, chopped

Place four crepes on baking sheet and sprinkle with cheese, one tablespoon peppers, tomatoes, and chicken strips. Place remaining four crepes on top. Top with remaining ingredients. Bake at 350 degrees for ten to fifteen minutes. Cut into wedges and serve.

225 calories per crepe
3.2 grams fat
11 grams carbohydrates
24 grams protein
Makes four servings

Chicken in Acorn Squash

This is a tasty and unique recipe. It is a pretty dish to serve, and the bottom layer of acorn squash pleases and surprises the palate greatly.

4 chicken breasts, cut into squares
2 acorn squash
1 red pepper, chopped
1 scallion, chopped
2 Italian tomatoes, chopped
pepper to taste

Ginger Sauce:

Combine in small bowl, 2 tablespoons dry sherry wine and 2 tablespoons low-sodium soy sauce. Add 3/4 cup low-sodium chicken broth, 1 tablespoon corn starch, 1 tablespoon brown sugar, and 1 teaspoon ground ginger.

Cut squash in half, scoop out seeds, and place face down in baking pan filled with 1/2 inch of water. Bake at 400 degrees for 40 minutes. About 15 minutes before squash is done, heat skillet coated with vegetable spray on medium high heat. Add chicken and cook for five minutes. Add pepper, scallion, tomatoes, and pepper, and cook for five minutes. Add ginger sauce and bring to a boil. Reduce heat and simmer for an additional five minutes. Spoon chicken mixture over squash halves and surround with wild rice.

202 calories per serving	30 grams carbohydrates	Makes four servings
6 grams fat	29 grams protein	

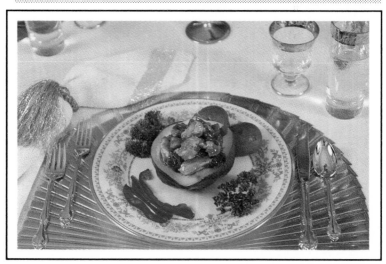

Low-Fat Shrimp Scampi

The flavor of shrimp scampi without all the fat found in the traditional recipe can be enjoyed by using intelligent low-fat substitutions. Serve with wild rice and a steamed vegetable for a quick meal.

1 pound uncooked, de-veined shrimp
2 scallions, chopped
3 tablespoons, chopped garlic
1/2 cup dry white wine
2 tablespoons lemon juice
pepper to taste
vegetable spray

Coat a large skillet with vegetable spray. Add scallions and garlic and saute over low heat for about ten minutes. Add shrimp and cook just until pink. Remove shrimp and keep warm. Add wine and lemon juice to skillet and simmer for three minutes. Season with pepper and pour over shrimp.

120 calories per 3 ounces of shrimp
1 gram fat
0.2 grams carbohydrates
23 grams protein
Makes four servings

Baked Shrimp

Dijon mustard and a dash of pepper sauce add great flavor to this baked shrimp dish without adding heavy oils for a sauce. Serve with rice or over pasta with Tomato-Basil Sauce (see recipe).

2 pounds large shrimp, shelled and de-veined
1/2 cup dry bread crumbs, Italian flavor
vegetable spray

Wine Mixture:
1/4 cup dry white wine
2 tablespoons fresh lemon juice
3 tablespoons garlic, minced
2 teaspoons fresh basil, chopped
1 teaspoon Worcestershire sauce
1/8 teaspoon hot pepper sauce
2 tablespoons Dijon mustard

Coat a large baking dish with vegetable spray. In another bowl, combine ingredients for the wine mixture and mix well. Remove 1/4 cup of the mixture and set aside. Add shrimp to baking dish and pour wine mixture over shrimp. Combine bread crumbs with reserved mixture and sprinkle over shrimp. Bake at 450 degrees for ten to fifteen minutes.

150 calories per 3 ounces of shrimp
1 gram fat
0.8 grams carbohydrates
23 grams protein
Makes four servings

Low-Fat, Low-Calorie Main Dishes

Sole Fillets with Lemon-Yogurt Sauce

The lemon yogurt sauce adds a tangy flavor to the fish and helps to keep it moist during cooking.

4 sole fillets
1/3 cup non-fat yogurt, plain
2 tablespoons lemon juice
1 tablespoon Dijon mustard
1 tablespoons horseradish

Place sole fillets in baking dish. In small bowl, blend yogurt, lemon juice, mustard, and horseradish. Spread mixture over fish. Cover and bake at 375 degrees for 15 minutes. Fish should flake easily with fork.

95 calories per fillet
1 gram fat
17 grams protein
0.2 grams carbohydrates
Makes four servings

Stuffed Flounder

This low-fat version of an elegant entree will please all seafood lovers.

8 flounder fillets
pepper
vegetable spray

Stuffing:
2 scallions, chopped
1 stalk celery, finely chopped
2 shallots, chopped
1/2 green pepper, chopped
2 tablespoons minced garlic
1 tablespoon whole wheat flour
1/2 cup dry white wine
1/2 cup skim milk
1/2 pound shrimp, boiled and chopped
1/2 pound lump crab meat, shredded
1/2 cup bread crumbs
2 tablespoons parsley
2 egg whites, lightly beaten
pepper to taste
cayenne pepper to taste

225 calories per fillet
2 grams fat
11 grams carbohydrates
23 grams protein
Makes four servings

Coat a large baking pan with vegetable spray. Spray the flounder fillets lightly, as well. Season with pepper. In a large skillet coated with vegetable spray, cook scallions, celery, shallots, green pepper, and garlic on medium heat until tender. Blend in flour. Remove from heat and add next six ingredients. Season to taste with black and cayenne peppers. To assemble, divide stuffing to top four fillets. Top with remaining fillets and press edges of fish together to seal. Cover and bake at 375 degrees for 25 minutes. Remove cover and bake an additional five minutes to brown lightly.

Love Those Carbohydrates

Our bodies must have carbohydrates to function properly. Carbohydrates provide the primary source of energy for all activity, both mental and physical. They are present in starches, sugars, fruits, vegetables, and grains. Learning to control carbohydrates can be tricky and difficult to understand.

The American diet has come to depend too heavily on the simple carbohydrates found in white sugar, white rice, and white flour. Foods made primarily with these are lacking in the vitamin B group. Sugar is essential in the diet. The brain burns sugar for its fuel. A lack of sugar can directly affect the ability to think and function. A diet too high in simple sugar begins a roller coaster existence.

Think of a normal American breakfast of coffee, sweet roll, or toast or doughnut or sweetened cereal. A sudden flush of energy is felt, because the sugar contained in this type of meal is simple and requires little from the body to break it up and convert it to energy. However, with no nutritional benefits, a short time later, energy levels diminish. The metabolism is out of balance. Hunger strikes, and fatigue is felt.

Sixty percent of each meal should contain complex carbohydrates which are rich in fiber, vitamins, and minerals. An over-consumption of carbohydrates will cause the body to store any excess as fat for later use as energy. Weight loss can't begin until fat reserves are depleted. These recipes are designed for nutritional value and fat content, and mainly for taste.

Flavored Couscous

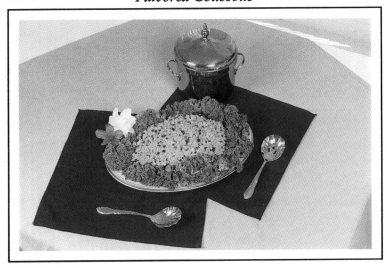

Love Those Carbohydrates

Fake Fettuccine Alfredo

Everyone seems to love fettuccine alfredo; however the waistline does not! There is a way to fake the flavor of this famous Italian dish, without the fat, by using the new flavored seasonings available. I discovered this one day eating a dish of plain pasta for lunch in our Sports Cafe. This recipe uses angel hair pasta formed into a mold, then sliced.

   1 package angel hair pasta
   2 cups water
   butter and sour cream flavored seasonings (by Molly
      McButter)

In tall saucepan, bring water to a boil and add pasta. Cook on high heat until all water is absorbed. Flip onto a plate and cut into pie wedges. Sprinkle with seasoned flavorings.

105 calories
1 gram fat
20 grams carbohydrates
4 grams protein
Makes six to eight servings

Love Those Carbohydrates

Spaghetti Squash Pancakes

Spaghetti squash makes a colorful, low-fat side dish. The squash can be baked whole in a regular oven or cut in half and microwaved. One squash yields five to seven cups of spaghetti squash for use in a variety of ways. Try something new for the family dinner! One pleasing way to serve this squash is for use in spicy, dinner pancakes. The flavor is unusual, low in fat, and tasty.

4 egg whites
3 cups cooked spaghetti squash
2 tablespoons ground ginger
2 scallions, chopped
vegetable spray

Pierce squash with fork in several places, and bake at 350 degrees for 45 minutes. Rotate and bake for 20 minutes longer. The squash can be microwaved. Cut squash in half and place cut side up in a safe, microwave dish. Add a small amount of water, cover, and microwave for 15 minutes, rotating every five minutes. Remove and let cool. Scrape out inside strands of squash with a fork. In a large bowl, beat egg whites with wire whisk. Add squash, ginger, and scallions. Mix gently. In a large skillet coated with vegetable spray, pour 1/4 cup of squash mixture into skillet. Space pancakes three inches apart. Cook two to three minutes, turn and cook two more minutes on other side. Serve with a low-sodium soy sauce on the side.

47 calories
3.2 grams fat
3.2 grams carbohydrates
1.4 grams protein
Makes four servings

Love Those Carbohydrates

Cold Rice Salad

This rice salad tastes best if refrigerated overnight before serving. Use a wild rice or rice pilaf mix. Do not add butter to the recipe! This dish works well for a buffet, because it is served at room temperature.

1 package wild rice mix, cooked and cooled slightly
1 pound sliced mushrooms
4 scallions, chopped fine
3 tablespoons red wine vinegar
1/2 teaspoon Dijon mustard
pepper to taste

Toss rice, mushrooms, and onions together in a large bowl. Combine remaining ingredients in small bowl and blend well. Pour over rice mixture and toss gently. Cover and let stand in the refrigerator overnight. Serve at room temperature.

200 calories per cup
0.6 grams fat
44 grams carbohydrates
4 grams protein
Makes four to six servings

Love Those Carbohydrates

Flavored Couscous

Couscous is a Moroccan pasta found in most grocer's rice section. Although a staple of the Mediterranean diet for centuries, couscous, only recently, has become popular with American cooks. It makes a nice change from rice, pasta, or potatoes. Flavored with chicken broth, this ethnic dish is tasty and low in fat.

1 box couscous
1 can low-sodium chicken broth
pepper

In saucepan, bring chicken broth to a boil, add couscous, and remove from heat. Cover and let stand for five minutes. Fluff with fork and season with pepper.

16 calories
0.2 grams fat
44 grams carbohydrates
4 grams protein
Makes four servings

Broccoli Baklava

Phyllo dough is a fat-free, thin Greek dough found in the grocer's freezer. It is easy to work with because it comes in flat sheets and can be manipulated. Spraying the dough with vegetable spray will keep it from breaking and will eliminate the need for butter. Other vegetables can be substituted for broccoli. Try asparagus!

2 tablespoons whole wheat flour
1/2 cup skim milk
2 scallions, chopped
1 8-ounce package non-fat cheddar cheese, shredded
6 egg whites
2 packages frozen, chopped broccoli
phyllo dough

Coat a casserole dish with vegetable spray. Stir flour and skim milk together until flour dissolves. In a large skillet coated with vegetable spray, saute onion for one minute. Add milk mixture and stir until thickened. Add cheese and broccoli. Remove from heat and stir in egg whites. Coat phyllo dough lightly with vegetable spray. In a manner similar to layering lasagne, layer dough and broccoli mixture. End with dough on top. Spray again with vegetable spray so top will brown. Bake at 325 degrees for 35 to 40 minutes. Cut into squares for serving.

117 calories
2 grams fat
18 grams carbohydrates
6 grams protein
Makes eight to ten servings

Love Those Carbohydrates

Stuffed Acorn Squash

Try offering squash once a week for dinner at home as a nice change from potatoes or pasta. I learned to enjoy squash as a child and love its flavor and texture. If you have never tried acorn squash, you are in for a treat! A cooking tip: Bake sweet potatoes or yams in the oven in the same manner white, baking potatoes are baked. This high heat method will release a carmelized sugar around the base of the potato.

4 acorn squash
6 sweet potatoes, washed and pierced once with fork
2 tablespoons honey
1/4 cup orange juice
1/2 teaspoon almond extract

Cut acorn squash in half. Place cut side down in baking pan and fill with 1/2 inch of water. Bake at 350 degrees for 45 minutes. Remove and turn squash side up and keep warm. Drain water. While squash is cooking, bake the sweet potatoes for one hour. Remove and peel skins. In large mixing bowl, whip sweet potatoes, honey, orange juice, and almond extract. Spoon or pipe into squash halves. Bake at 350 degrees for 20 minutes.

280 calories
1 gram fat
41 grams carbohydrates
7 grams protein
Makes eight servings

Love Those Carbohydrates

Twice-Baked Potatoes

These twice-baked potatoes are very popular and satisfying, without the extra fat and calories found in the traditional recipe. I bake an extra potato with each recipe to make extra full potatoes when stuffing the shells, and in case a potato shell is damaged. The potatoes are so tasty, it's hard to believe they are low in fat!

6 large baking potatoes, washed, dried, & pierced with a fork
1 carton non-fat yogurt, plain
1 8-ounce package non-fat cheddar cheese, shredded
2 scallions, chopped
2 teaspoons onion powder
1 tablespoon salt substitute
pepper to taste
paprika

Bake potatoes at 425 degrees for at least one hour. Cooking the potatoes at a high temperature will give a crispy crust with moist potatoes inside. Slice potatoes in half, lengthwise. Scoop out the inside of each potato carefully, making certain not to damage the shells. Place in baking pan. In large bowl, whip potatoes, yogurt, scallions, onion powder, salt substitute, and pepper with an electric hand mixer. Add cheese and whip at low speed. Spoon potato mixture into shells, and sprinkle with paprika. Bake at 375 degrees for 20 to 25 minutes or until potatoes are golden brown.

110 calories
1 gram fat
22 grams carbohydrates
2 grams protein
Makes ten servings

Love Those Carbohydrates

Low-Fat Potato Salad

Most potato salad is the too-fat version served in most restaurants, which must avoided. Potato salad lovers will enjoy this low-fat version for picnics, parties, or any family gathering. And this recipe is quick and easy because the potatoes are microwaved while the rest of the ingredients are being assembled.

3 large potatoes, washed and pierced once with fork
3/4 cup non-fat Miracle Whip or mayonnaise
1 celery stalk, finely chopped
1 scallion, finely chopped
3-1/2 tablespoons mustard
pepper to taste

Microwave potatoes on high for five minutes. Rotate and cook for an additional five minutes. Remove and let cool. Peel and cut potatoes into squares. Transfer potatoes to a bowl and add remaining ingredients. Mix well. Sprinkle with paprika for extra flavor and color. Chill thoroughly before serving.

95 calories per cup
0.6 grams fat
22 grams carbohydrates
2 grams protein
Makes four servings

Love Those Carbohydrates

Quick Potato Casserole

This quick casserole can be made with instant mashed potatoes or from mashed potatoes made from scratch. Either way, this dish is a winner!

4 egg whites
4 cups instant mashed potatoes, cooked
1 8-ounce package non-fat cheddar cheese, shredded
1 scallion, finely chopped
1 teaspoon onion powder
1/2 teaspoon salt substitute
paprika
vegetable spray

Coat a three quart casserole dish with vegetable spray. Using an electric mixer, beat egg whites into potatoes. Blend in cheese, scallions, onion powder, and salt substitute. Carefully spoon potato mixture into casserole dish and sprinkle with paprika. Bake uncovered for 25 minutes or until golden brown.

80 calories per serving
0.6 grams fat
23 grams carbohydrates
3 grams protein
Makes four to five servings

Love Those Carbohydrates

Low-Fat Noodle Kugal

Noodle Kugal is a traditional, Jewish holiday dish, which is usually very fattening. This recipe version continues the tasty tradition without the fat and calories by using yellow and black raisins for distinctive flavoring.

1 package angel hair noodles
1/2 cup black raisins
1/2 cup yellow raisins
2 tablespoons ground cinnamon
1 tablespoon lemon peel
6 egg whites
vegetable spray

Cook noodles according to package directions and drain. In a large mixing bowl, add cooked noodles and remaining ingredients. Mix well. Pour into baking pan coated with vegetable spray. Bake at 350 degrees for 40 minutes. Turn oven to broil, and heat for five additional minutes until top is golden brown.

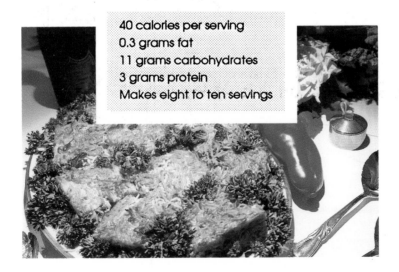

40 calories per serving
0.3 grams fat
11 grams carbohydrates
3 grams protein
Makes eight to ten servings

Love Those Carbohydrates

Low-Fat Potato Pancakes

Potato pancakes have long been served in Jewish homes. This low-fat version will measure up in flavor to the traditional recipe.

> 4 potatoes, fully baked & peeled or 1 bag fresh, frozen
>   potatoes
> 3/4 cup Italian bread crumbs
> 4 egg whites
> 1 cup skim milk
> 1/2 onion, chopped
> 1 teaspoon salt substitute
> 1 teaspoon onion powder
> vegetable spray

In a blender, combine all ingredients and blend until smooth. Heat skillet coated with vegetable spray on high heat. Pour 1/3 cup of batter for each pancake and cook for three minutes on each side or until golden brown. Repeat until all of the batter has been used.

35 calories per pancake
0.2 grams fat
11 grams carbohydrates
2 grams protein
Makes six to eight servings

Love Those Carbohydrates

Potato Pie

This quick side dish can be made even more quickly by using fresh, frozen potato products now available in the grocer's frozen vegetable section. Potatoes can be baked ahead of time to make preparation faster when using fresh baking potatoes.

3 cups frozen potatoes or 3 large baking potatoes, skins
    peeled and cut into squares
10 egg whites
3 scallions, chopped
1/2 cup chopped green pepper
1 8-ounce carton non-fat yogurt, plain
pepper to taste
vegetable spray

Coat pie plate with vegetable spray. Whisk egg whites, scallions, and black pepper in large bowl. Add potatoes, green pepper, and yogurt. Stir well. Pour into pie plate and bake at 350 degrees for one hour and 15 minutes. Cut into pie wedges to serve.

180 calories
1 gram fat
27 grams carbohydrates
6 grams protein
Makes six to eight servings

Love Those Carbohydrates

Low-Fat Yorkshire Pudding

Yorkshire pudding was always popular around my house when I was growing up, and my mother added yellow raisins for extra flavor. The corner pieces were eaten first, because of their extra crisp, golden brown crunch! The flavor of this traditional pudding can be duplicated using low-fat substitutions.

2 egg whites
1/2 cup all-purpose flour
1/2 cup skim milk
1 teaspoon sugar
1/3 cup yellow raisins
1/3 cup black raisins
butter flavored vegetable spray

In blender, combine egg whites, flour, milk, and sugar. Mix well. Stir in raisins. Coat a ten inch, oven-proof skillet with vegetable spray. Heat over high heat. Immediately pour batter into skillet, and bake in oven at 425 degrees for 25 minutes. Serve warm.

60 calories per serving
1.5 grams fat
3.4 grams protein
9.8 grams carbohydrates
Makes four to six servings

Sweet Endings

Sweet Endings...Without The Guilt

I love dessert, but don't we all! There is a way to have dessert without the calories, sugar, fat, or guilt! Use cocoa powder instead of chocolate. Reduce sugar, butter, and flour amounts. Use egg whites instead of whole eggs. Ready-made crepes can be used for many quick dessert ideas. Experiment! Low-fat cooking substitution will soon become easy and natural. Try these recipes and think substitution. Create your own version of traditional family recipes using my ideas and your talent!

Fresh Fruit Pizza

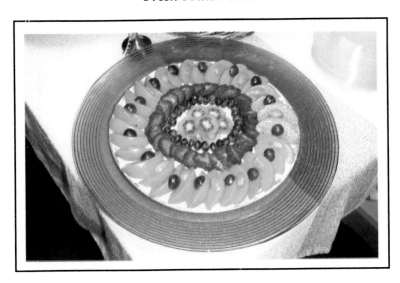

Sweet Endings

Pumpkin Cake with Neufatchel Frosting

This low-fat pumpkin cake is fun to serve for Halloween or Thanksgiving. The cake has a wonderful flavor with or without the suggested frosting.

8 egg whites
2 cups all-purpose flour
2 teaspoons baking soda
1 teaspoon ground cloves
2 teaspoons cinnamon
1/2 teaspoon ground ginger
1/2 teaspoon nutmeg
1/2 cup sugar
2 tablespoons honey
1 can packed pumpkin

Sift flour with baking soda. Add all spices. With electric mixer at high speed, beat egg whites, sugar, and honey until light and fluffy (about five minutes). Gradually add pumpkin to flour mixture until combined. Pour into ungreased nine inch tube pan, and bake at 350 degrees for one hour. Completely cook cake in pan before removing.

Neufatchel Frosting:
1 package Neufatchel cream cheese
1 tablespoon vanilla extract
1/4 cup sugar

Microwave cheese for 30 seconds until soft. Remove and mix with vanilla extract and sugar until smooth and creamy. Frost Pumpkin Cake!

180 calories
3 grams fat
3 grams protein
23 grams carbohydrates
Makes ten to twelve servings

118

Sweet Endings

Gingerbread with Lemon Sauce

Gingerbread is an all-time favorite dessert both to taste and smell. The lemon sauce adds a tart topping without the extra calories and fat. This recipe makes a wonderful healthy, homemade gift during the holidays.

1 cup all-purpose flour
1/4 cup sugar
2 teaspoons pumpkin pie spice
2 egg whites
2 tablespoons molasses
1/2 cup hot water
1 teaspoon baking soda
vegetable spray

Combine flour, sugar, and pumpkin pie spice in a mixing bowl. In another small bowl, combine egg whites and molasses. Set aside. In a third bowl, combine water and baking soda. Add molasses mixture and water mixture to the flour mixture and stir well. Pour batter into an eight inch baking pan that has been coated with vegetable spray. Bake at 450 degrees for 20 minutes. Cool slightly. Cut into squares and top with lemon sauce.

Lemon Sauce:
3 tablespoons sugar
2 teaspoons corn starch
1/2 teaspoon lemon rind
2 tablespoons lemon juice

Combine all ingredients in a saucepan and cook over medium heat until thickened.

120 calories per serving
1 gram fat
25 grams carbohydrates
3.3 protein
Makes eight to ten servings

Fresh Fruit Pizza

Fresh fruit pizza has become a favorite with customers at our Sports Cafe. It is different, elegant, and wonderful! The crust is made with flour and egg whites and covered with Neufatchel cheese (1/3 less fat than regular cream cheese), then flavored with almond extract and topped with fresh fruit. Use fruits which will not discolor. Canned peaches and mandarin oranges in light syrup work well drained. Fresh strawberries, kiwi, raspberries, and red or green grapes make a beautiful pizza.

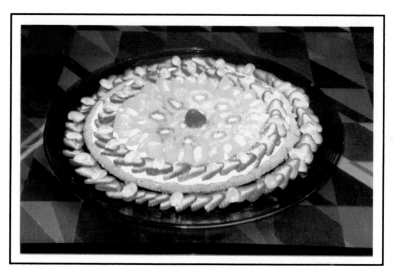

Pizza Crust:
1/2 cup extra light margarine, room temperature or soften
   in microwave for 20 seconds
1 cup water
1/4 cup sugar
2 egg whites
1 teaspoon vanilla extract
2 cups all-purpose flour
1/2 teaspoon baking soda
1/2 teaspoon cream of tartar
vegetable spray

Using an electric mixer, cream margarine. Add sugar and beat until light and fluffy. Add egg whites, vanilla extract, water and beat well. In another bowl, combine flour, baking soda, and cream of tartar. Stir into creamed mixture. Shape into a ball, cover, and refrigerate for one hour. Preheat over to 375 degrees. Spray pizza pan with vegetable spray. Roll out dough to fit pan. Bake for 15 to 20 minutes or until golden brown. Remove and let cool.

Frosting:

1 8-ounce package Neufatchel cheese
3 tablespoons sugar
1-1/2 teaspoons almond extract

Microwave Neufatchel cheese for 30 seconds. Add sugar and almond extract and mix well. Spread on pizza crust to within 1/8 inch of edge. Top with sliced fruit.

110 calories per slice
3 grams fat
2 grams protein
24 grams carbohydrates
Makes ten to twelve servings

Sweet Endings

Chocolate Raspberry Cheesecake
with Raspberry Sauce

Yes, you really can make a rich and creamy, low-fat cheesecake! This recipe can be adapted by using other flavors found in typical cheesecake recipes like amaretto, lemon, or orange by using extracts or liqueurs.

1/2 cup low-fat, ricotta cheese
1 large carton plain or vanilla non-fat yogurt
3 egg whites
1/4 cup sugar
1/3 cup chocolate raspberry cocoa powder
2 tablespoons flour
2 teaspoons vanilla extract
1/3 cup chocolate wafers, crushed in blender

Place yogurt in cheese cloth and let drain overnight in a strainer set in a bowl in the refrigerator. With an electric mixer, blend egg whites and sugar for five minutes. Add ricotta cheese, drained yogurt, cocoa powder, flour, and vanilla. Spray spring form pan with vegetable spray. Press chocolate wafer crumbs to the bottom of the pan evenly. Pour cake mixture into pan. Bake at 325 degrees for 50 minutes. Cool in oven, door open, oven off. Top with fresh fruit. Strawberries or raspberries look wonderful!

Raspberry Sauce:

This sauce can be made quickly to serve on the side or on top of cheesecake. Use two packages frozen, unsweetened raspberries, thawed. Press through sieve into saucepan and bring to a boil Add one teaspoon raspberry liqueur, reduce heat, and simmer until sauce thickens. Cool.

160 calories
5 grams fat per slice
11 grams carbohydrates
2 grams protein
Makes eight to ten servings

Orange Chiffon Cheesecake

This is another great, low-fat recipe for cheesecake lovers. Garnish with orange slices and graham cracker crumbs for a special dessert.

1 cup graham cracker crumbs
1 pkg. gelatin
6 egg whites
1/2 cup skim milk
1/3 cup low-fat, ricotta cheese
1/3 cup orange juice
2 tablespoons orange liqueur
1 envelope dessert topping mix
2 tablespoons sugar

Coat a spring form pan with vegetable spray, and press graham cracker crumbs to pan. Set in refrigerator. In small bowl, soften gelatin in 1/4 cup water. In medium saucepan, combine skim milk, ricotta cheese, orange juice, sugar, and softened gelatin. Stir well over medium heat for 20 minutes. Do not boil mixture. Remove from heat and chill until partially set. Prepare topping mix, using skim milk, and fold into gelatin mixture. In a large bowl, beat egg whites until stiff peaks form. Fold into gelatin mixture. Pour into pan and chill until set and ready to serve.

120 calories per serving
4 grams fat
Makes eight to ten servings

Sweet Endings

Spreadable Fruit Crepes

Didn't prepare dessert but your sweet tooth needs a quick fix? Instead of reaching for the cookie jar, try this recipe idea. It will satisfy your need for something sweet with very little fat. These crepes are quick and easy and can be prepared for one or one hundred!

1 ready-made crepe
1 tablespoon spreadable fruit, any flavor
powdered sugar, optional

Place crepe on a microwave dish. Spoon spreadable fruit down the middle. Fold over edges and flatten. Microwave for 10 seconds on high and remove. Sprinkle with powdered sugar and serve.

132 calories
1 gram fat
2 grams protein
4.3 grams carbohydrates
Makes one serving

Sweet Endings

Chocolate Raspberry Fondue with Fresh Fruit

This recipe calls for chocolate raspberry cocoa powder which is available in the gourmet section of most grocery stores. By using cocoa powder instead of chocolate squares, the fat content is reduced to one gram per serving. Serve with your favorite fruit. Strawberries, raspberries, peaches, banana chunks, and orange sections all work well for this fondue.

    3 tablespoons chocolate raspberry cocoa powder
    3 tablespoons brown sugar
    1-1/2 teaspoons cornstarch
    1/2 cup water
    3 tablespoons honey
    1-1/2 teaspoons vanilla extract
    pinch of salt

Place all ingredients in a saucepan and mix thoroughly over medium heat. Bring to a low boil. Serve in a fondue pot.

19.8 calories per 3 tablespoons
1 gram fat
2.1 gram protein
18 grams carbohydrates
Recipe yields two cups

Sweet Endings

Strawberry Souffle

This souffle is served hot with a yogurt and vanilla topping. Use spreadable fruit and egg whites to create this low-fat, elegant dessert.

8 egg whites, at room temperature
1/4 teaspoon cream of tartar
1 tablespoon lemon juice
2 teaspoons grated lemon rind
1 jar spreadable fruit, strawberry or raspberry
1/4 cup all-purpose flour
2 tablespoons sugar
vegetable spray

Combine flour and sugar and set aside in small bowl. In another bowl, combine spreadable fruit, lemon juice, and lemon rind. Using a hand mixer, add flour mixture to fruit mixture, and beat at low speed until smooth. In another bowl, beat egg whites and cream of tartar until stiff peaks form. Gently add one quarter of the egg white mixture to the fruit mixture to lighten it. Then add remaining egg white mixture and pour into souffle dish coated with vegetable spray. Bake at 400 degrees for 10 to 12 minutes or until the top is golden brown. Serve immediately with plain, non-fat yogurt flavored with vanilla extract.

98 calories per serving
1 gram fat
3 grams protein
32 grams carbohydrates
Makes six servings

Sweet Endings

Bags of Apples

This dessert tastes, smells, and looks wonderful! It's like apple pie without the extra fat, calories, or guilt. Allow one apple per person. This recipe can easily be doubled or adjusted to the number of people being served.

1 package phyllo dough, refrigerate until ready to use
4 apples, cut into squares
2 tablespoons lemon juice
3 tablespoons brown sugar
2 tablespoons black raisins
2 tablespoons yellow raisins
1 tablespoon arrowroot
1-1/2 teaspoon ground cinnamon
1 teaspoon ground nutmeg
1 teaspoon ground cloves
vegetable spray

Combine apples and lemon juice, and mix well until all apples are coated with juice. In a small bowl, combine brown sugar, raisins, arrowroot, cinnamon, nutmeg, and cloves. Stir well and combine with the apples. Place three sheets of pastry dough on a cookie sheet and spray with vegetable spray. Spoon 3/4 cup of apple mixture into center of dough and bring up edges. Pinch dough together, leaving extra phyllo at the top. Spray dough again with vegetable spray. Repeat with remaining ingredients. Bake at 350 degrees for 35 to 40 minutes.

Tip: If you like well-done apples, microwave apple mixture for one minute before placing in phyllo dough.

198 calories
4.3 grams fat
39.8 grams carbohydrates
2.5 grams protein
Makes six servings

Low-Fat Chocolate Chip Cookies

This cookie uses 1/2 the fat and 1/2 the chips of the original recipe.

1/2 cup sugar
1/4 cup brown sugar
1/4 cup margarine, softened
1 teaspoon vanilla
2 egg whites
1 cup flour
1/2 teaspoon baking soda
1/2 cup mini chips

Mix sugars, margarine, vanilla and egg white in a large bowl. Stir in flour and baking soda. Stir in Mini-chips. Drop dough onto ungreased cookie sheet. Bake at 375 degrees for 8-10 minutes.

75 calories
2 grams fat
14 grams carbohydrates
1 grams protein